ONE
BARBER'S
STORY

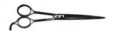

From Sicily to America

ONE
BARBER'S
STORY

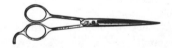

From Sicily to America

Pasquale Spagnuolo

ST. MARTIN'S PRESS ☒ NEW YORK

Design by Sara Stemen

The author and publisher are grateful for permission to reprint
the following:
"Mr. Know-How." Reprinted by permission; © 1951, 1979. The
New Yorker Magazine, Inc.
"Ties." Reprinted by permission; © 1967. The New Yorker
Magazine, Inc.

LIBRARY OF CONGRESS CATALOGING-IN-PUBLICATION DATA
Spagnuolo, Pasquale.
    One barber's story :   from Sicily to America   /
Pasquale Spagnuolo.
        p.   cm.
    "A Thomas Dunne book."
    ISBN 0-312-11872-4
    1. Spagnuolo, Pasquale.   2. Italian Americans—New York
(N.Y.)—Biography.   3. Barbers—New York (N.Y.)—
Biography.   4. New York (N.Y.)—Biography.   I. Title.
F128.9.I8S63   1995
646.7′24′092—dc20
[B]   94-48483
                                                                              CIP

First Edition: April 1995
10 9 8 7 6 5 4 3 2 1

I dedicate this book to my wife, Connie. During her illness with Alzheimer's and Parkinson's, she was sedated by eighteen pills a day, and I was alone. To occupy my time and not feel sorry for myself, I wrote this book, after jotting down notes for more than twenty years. While I was writing, I also devoted much time to my mandolin, composing the mazurka "My Connie."

MY CONNIE
MAZURKA
BY Pasquale Spagnuolo

Preface

I am a Sicilian immigrant who spent his life perfecting the craft of barbering. For many years I was the proud co-owner of the Arcade Barber Shop. This book tells my story.

Many Sicilians became tradesmen, carpenters, shoemakers, tailors, and barbers. Nearly 95 percent of the Italian immigrants to the United States were Sicilians. Most of them had a "five-year plan" to save enough money to return home and buy land, or a house, or both. Many of the women—and some of the men—worked in sweatshop clothing factories. The men were usually cutters, and the women, expert with needles, produced the finished clothes. Work was arduous: ten hours long, six days a week; Sundays they worked only five hours.

Most Sicilian immigrants were manual laborers, usually getting their jobs through friends. Many never had time to learn English. Employers suspected that when their workers had saved enough, they would go home. These were the days of the real "minorities," long before social services, pensions, and relief checks for the out-of-work. Medical care was provided to no one, and Medicare was many decades in the future. Not until the mid-1920s, when the garment workers formed a union, did working conditions begin to improve.

Once in America, families from the same Sicilian towns lived near one another, visiting on Sunday evenings and reminiscing about their hometowns and their friends and relatives there. They talked about their sacrifices and how much more they would have to give. The families helped and depended on one another and often found jobs for new immigrants. In the old country, there was little chance to possess any more than you were born with. Nonetheless, people lived happily.

I can remember being reminded of family goals—money accumulated and plans and dreams for using it. Such decisions were always being discussed and debated. How much money should we send home? How much more money did we need to return home to Sicily?

This memoir recounts the history of Licodia Eubea, my hometown, my family history, and interesting small-game hunting stories with special hunting dogs. I come from a family of hunters. The sport provided both exercise and fresh air, which were a needed relief after working indoors.

I also relate my Golden Rules on serving the public as an employer and as an employee, the unique method of advertising that gave us immediate results, and many intimate stories of clients (some very well known) during my fifty-five years of barbering, a trade I was proud of. I always tried to provide the ultimate in service and workmanship, and I include stories about perfecting our massaging and scalp treatment shampooing, the ins and outs of barbering, and my special technique for getting clients to sell services to themselves with supersuccess.

Writing this book has revived many pleasant memories. There are stories of certain special people, some of whom I still keep in touch with. I was fortunate to have them as friends.

ONE
BARBER'S
STORY

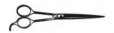

From Sicily to America

1

LICODIA Eubea was originally built by Greeks from Calcidesi di Eubea who explored Sicily about 730 B.C. Landing at what is now Messina, they went south along the sea to the town of Taormina, proceeded to Catania, then on to Lentini. Mount Etna and its volcano could be seen from all these places. As the Greeks proceeded south and moved inland, they discovered virgin lands and were amazed at the quality of the soil.

At last they came upon a mountain, some two thousand feet above sea level. Realizing that a town here would command a view of the surrounding countryside, the Greeks built one halfway up the south side of the heights. They named it Eubea, after their home in Greece. The lands around the mountain had water for irrigation and were fertile, making them exceptional for growing vegetables. Eubea, along with Catania, Imera, and Lentini, was ruled by the laws of Carando, in Greece.

In time, Eubea began to prosper. Her wealth

JOHNNY CARSON

Johnny came to the Arcade Barber Shop for nearly ten years, until his fame took him to the West Coast. When he came in for his usual haircut and manicure, he never had much to say and did not like being recognized. It was difficult not to be recognized, as the shop was fifty by twenty feet with windows on two sides. There were often ten to fifteen people waiting for Johnny Carson's autograph, or to shake his hand as he went out into the lobby of the building. He obliged their enthusiasm but detested it. One day, having had enough of his aggressive fans, he called to have Jerry Grimaldi, who usually cut his hair, sent to his office with a manicurist. Jerry continued this until Carson went to California.

In 1986, my wife, Connie, and I went to Burbank, California, for a two-month vacation to visit Connie's sister, Josie. While we were there, I called Johnny Carson's secretary, requesting five tickets to his show. She said that she

reached the point that neighboring Siracusa's leader, the tyrant Gelone (who was well fortified, having spent many years strengthening his position), decided to attack Eubea by surprise. He destroyed the small town, taking some of the inhabitants prisoner and bringing them to Siracusa. Others were sold as slaves. The few who escaped hid in caves.

Hundreds of years later, Eubea was still in ruins. In this period, a band of dispossessed Italians, most from an Arab background and calling themselves "Saracini" were sent to Sicily by the Italian Senate to find homes for themselves, only to discover deplorable conditions. But when the Saracini found the ruins of Eubea, with its fertile land and its picturesque views, they decided to build a town. They chose the top of the mountain, ignoring the ruins of Eubea hundreds of feet below. They named the settlement Licodia, from the word *lykos* (wolf), since there were many wolves in the territory. The new flag depicted a wolf.

As years passed, Licodia slowly regained Eubea's surrounding counties and began to prosper, growing grain, olives, beans, grapes, almonds, oranges, lemons, tangerines, and abundant vegetables. Her tobacco crops were famous throughout Sicily as the best grown anywhere.

In the early twelfth century, the Saracini built a fortress *(castello)* with five turrets just south of the center of town to protect Licodia against attack. The *castello* overlooked great distances on all sides and was always ready to repel enemies.

Licodia was rebuilt in the time of Augustus, about 63 B.C. to A.D. 14, who started building first at the top of the southern side of the mountain, calling it Santa Lucia, and in later years continued building farther up, along the east side. The peak stood out above the town about a quarter mile wide, half a mile long, and three hundred feet high.

wasn't allowed to give more than three tickets but would call back. She called later, informing me that there would be five tickets in my name at the box office. She added a message from Johnny saying he hadn't forgotten the Arcade Barber Shop. Carson asked for my home address and sent me an autographed photograph.

Don Utero Santapau bought the title of prince of Palazzolo (a very small town nearby), making his residence in Licodia's *castello.*

The Santapaus dominated Licodia for nearly 250 years, until 1693, when an earthquake destroyed the *castello* and its turrets, killing about one thousand people. With it went the Santapaus, leaving only the name: "Castello Santapao." One hundred years later, Licodia added its original name, Eubea, to its current name, unofficially calling itself Licodia Eubea.

After the earthquake there was much digging for treasure in the castle, as the Santapaus had been very wealthy. Much treasure was found, and digging continued until the early nineteenth century, when the Italian government declared Santapao Castle a state monument, forbidding any more digging and building a road to the castle grounds for tourists.

MOE BEHRMAN, A FINE GENTLEMAN

I shaved Moe Behrman for more than twenty years, every day except Sunday. Moe was in partnership with his older brother, Harry, in an accounting firm at 535 Fifth Avenue; a younger brother, Sam, was a playwright. During the summer, Moe took his family to Asbury Park on weekends. He was an unusually kind and generous man who happened to have the strongest and most difficult gray beard to shave. He continually complained that on his Asbury Park weekends he never got a clean shave.

I explained that the price of a shave was half that of a haircut, but it took at least the same time. If a customer came in only for a shave, unless he was a regular client, barbers usually gave him a bad shave so that he would never come back. I suggested that next time, instead of the usual 15¢ tip, which was average in the late 1930s, as he sat down he tell the barber that he had lapses of memory and would

Following is writing found on a wall in one of the castle's underground dungeons:

How cold is this dungeon! It's like ice
With water seeping through all the walls
It's God's will that I embrace
The pains that I must absorb, from hour to hour
But if I live, Revenge I will have
With lead I will aim
And if I miss I will cut off my arm
Condemning myself on the spot

Very few families actually lived on their farms in Licodia. The men "commuted" to their farms daily, usually as much as two hours each way, by donkey, horse, or mule. The less fortunate walked, leaving their homes at 4:00 A.M. Licodiesi women never worked the fields alongside their husbands. The women were busy tending their children, washing clothes, sewing, cooking, shopping for food in the town market for anything they didn't produce on their land, and bringing three or four large clay jugs to the town's water pumps. People in better circumstances paid local women to get water for them; some even could afford servants to do it. Many times fights resulted when one woman put her jugs ahead of someone else's.

Licodia Eubea has a breathtaking command of the surrounding countryside. To the south one can see the Mediterranean Sea; from the east and west there are views of farmlands dotted with orange, tangerine, and lemon groves and numerous wheat fields. To the north rises Mt. Etna. On a clear night—which is most of the time—one can see the cities of Caltagirone and Vittoria, and the towns of Lentini, Comiso, Palazzolo and Grammichele, glittering with lights that seem to sparkle like stars.

The weather is ideal most of the year. July and August are very warm but pleasantly dry. The winter has a short rainy season that comes around January. And snow is such a novelty that children run out with pots to catch the flakes.

My maternal grandfather, Giuseppe Vassallo, was a descendant of the celebrated Emperor Constantine XI (Palaeologus) of Constantinople. Two of the emperor's sons went to Sicily, one to the town of Noto and the other to Palermo. The emperor ordered the name Paelogo to be changed to Vassallo. A second generation, now Vassallo, made their home in Licodia Eubea.

Our family seat, the Palazzo Vassallo, was built in the early 1700s and still stands in excellent condition. It has a Vassallo family crest over the entrance, reading *In Hoc Signo Vinces*. The original Pallazzo Vassallo had sixteen rooms on one floor, the smallest twenty-five feet square. Its domed ceilings were made of pumice, designed to keep heat in and cold out. In the

like to tip him beforehand. Then give him $1.

The coming Monday morning, Moe came to see me before going to the office. He grabbed me, hugging and kissing me, saying that I had made his weekends happy. From then on, he raised my shaving tip to 25¢ and the haircut tip to $1.

MY ADVERTISING SECRET

The Arcade Barber Shop was in the middle of the arcade in 25 West Forty-third Street, which went through to Forty-fourth Street. With no barbershop signs of any kind on the exterior of the building, my partner, Angelo Copertino, and I decided to do some advertising to let people know where we were. We decided to bring flyers and matchbooks in person to office buildings in our area. This was very hard work for us, going office to office in fifty- or sixty-story buildings, starting at the top and working our way down using stairways from floor to floor.

After doing this for a few years with very little result, I noticed that most clients coming in through the advertisements were new people moving into the area. Ninety-nine percent of our efforts in distributing flyers was a waste, as most people had been there for years and already had a barber. I had the idea of advertising only to new tenants coming into a

four corners of each room, where the dome met the yard-thick walls, stood beautiful sculptures.

Salvatore Vassallo, my great-uncle, willed the palazzo to his son Mario. Mario remained single until he was sixty, when his housekeeper, Donna Concetta, after many years in his employ, became his wife, although everyone suspected that they had lived as man and wife for a long time. Shortly after his father's death, Mario made four apartments of four rooms each out of the sixteen rooms in the palazzo. He kept the larger two apartments, which fronted the main entrance on Via Mugnos, and sold the two that fronted a back street, Via Corollo. It was very easy to divide the four apartments, as the palazzo possessed two large entrances. Each apartment had similar stairways with some twenty steps. In the middle of the building, there was an opening about forty feet square.

The two apartments fronting Via Corollo he sold with no rights to the two basements. These cellars were on the street level, each with about twenty-foot ceilings. Both had doors so large that a horse and buggy, or car, could drive in. Mario was a veterinarian and he used one basement apartment for operations on animals.

The apartment next to his remained empty because he was afraid of being robbed. He was a loner who suspected that everyone was after his money.

My grandfather, Giuseppe Vassallo, died in 1893. He left his wife, Cristina, with six children (two boys and four girls), but he left her in very comfortable circumstances with a lot of property. He was a shoemaker with a shop in the piazza where the Church Madrice had stood since 1621. My grandmother Cristina was a tiny woman, but she was very shrewd and capable. She managed the lands until her two sons, Nunzio and Francesco, were old enough to assume responsibility.

They followed in their father's footsteps, becoming shoemakers and reopening the old cobbler shop. Their father had taught them the trade. After they married, with their dowries and their wives' dowries, they lived very comfortably, so comfortably, in fact, that they practically opened the shop only on rainy days. They either went hunting during the season, or supervised the men who worked their lands. After the evening meal, they reopened the shop to meet with the leaders of the town to air views on current political issues be-

building. I approached Ronnie Rosenfeld, a client of our barber Vito Nobile, who was a top advertising executive with Doyle Dane Bernbach. Ronnie agreed to help us write a letter to people moving into the neighborhood:

Arcade Barber Shop
25 West 43rd Street
NYC 10036

Dear Mr. ———,

Moving into a new neighborhood is, at best, an exhausting experience. There are many details to attend to. Like opening a new bank account, finding a garage to park your car, someone to deliver your morning coffee. A few good restaurants that prepare food the way you like it.

Unfortunately, we can't help you with any of those things. But when it comes to taking care of your hair—we're experts.

Our eight barbers and two manicurists invite you to visit the Arcade Barber Shop, located in the main lobby of 25 West 43rd Street and 28 West 44th Street.

Isn't it nice to know that

there is a barber shop in your neighborhood—where you can be sure of courteous, efficient and friendly service?

Make a note of our number—Bryant 9-8283. When you have a few moments to spare, a quick phone call will insure you of an appointment with anyone on our staff.

Welcome to the neighborhood—and good luck in your new location. We hope to have the opportunity to serve you soon.

Very cordially yours,

Pat and Angelo
Co-Owners

We had five thousand letters made, four thousand starting with "Dear" and one thousand with "Dear Sir." I went to all the large office buildings within one block of our building that had no barbershops and approached the elevator operator. Introducing myself as the owner of the Arcade Barber Shop, I gave him a $10 bill and told him he would get another $10 each time he notified me of a new

hind closed doors and shutters, just as their father had done. Both brothers were well respected. My mother, Vincenza Vassallo, was the youngest of the six children. She was born on December 5, 1891.

My father, Francesco Spagnuolo, was born on July 2, 1889. He was the son of Pasquale Spagnuolo and Angela Pepi. My father had a sister, Giuseppa, and a stepbrother, Nunzio, a son of my grandfather's second wife.

My grandfather Pasquale was a farmer who worked his own lands, hiring help when necessary. He was so expert in judging horses, mules, and donkeys that he was always in demand to buy or sell animals, for a fee. He was also a supersalesman. This quality came in handy in making his three proposals of marriage (he was a widower twice).

My father showed a lot of potential in school, and his ambition was to go to college to obtain a degree. Unfortunately, my grandfather didn't share his objective; he wanted one member of his family to become a priest. Therefore, my father went into a monastery to study for the priesthood. When he was ordained a priest, my grandfather's face radiated with pride as his son served his first Mass in Licodia Eubea. My grandfather had notified everyone in town, and the church was packed. All present offered their congratulations to my father and grandfather. The happy event ended on a sad note, though. When everyone had left and the two were alone, my father said to my grandfather, "I will never say Mass again and make a mockery of the Catholic religion. I refuse to live a lie." My grandfather was furious, saying, "Then you will come with me and work on the farm." My father replied, "Gladly." He was very pleased with the outcome and faithfully attended Mass every Sunday.

One Sunday during Mass, my father caught the eye of my mother. From then on, every Sunday, he walked with friends about one hundred feet behind my mother, her mother, her brother, and his brother's wife on the way to church. During Mass they continued to eye each other. He began to take a great liking to Vincenza, but it was not acceptable for a daughter of a shoemaker (especially Giuseppe Vassallo's daughter) to marry a farmer. More important, her two brothers, Francesco and Nunzio, had informed my father that they didn't want him following them on their way to church anymore. Any thoughts he had about her, he should

tenant moving into the building.

When I was told of a new tenant moving in, I would visit that company's receptionist and hand her one of our "Dear Sir" letters. I would introduce myself and tell her I was sure the men in the office, being new in the area, would appreciate knowing about my first-class barbershop. While talking, I would take a small package (worth about $5) out of my pocket and give it to her, saying, "This is for your trouble." Unless it was a small firm, she would give me back the package, saying that she was not allowed to accept it.

I would give her back the package and ask if she could get me a list of the personnel in the office. She usually would bring it to the shop later. Upon receiving the list, I would insert men's names in my "Dear" letters. I never sent letters to more than fifteen out of one hundred names a day. I wanted to keep it from looking like an advertising drive.

The result was very successful. Usually on the day the letter was received, one person would call for an appointment or come in to see the shop on his lunch hour. They then would come two and three at a time, introducing themselves, telling us that they would be in soon. Most had visited their old barber shortly before moving. Rarely two or three months went by without a new tenant moving into one of these buildings, making our shop busy and successful, with all eight chairs working and an additional manicurist. To have three manicurists and eight barbers was a rarity. Usually there were only one or two.

forget, or they would see to it that he did. My mother also had noticed what was going on and had begun to like him. She knew of his past in the priesthood. Consequently she turned down many proposals of marriage from well-to-do young men. Her brothers chided her that if she didn't change her mind she would end up a spinster.

The Spagnuolos and the Vassallos had mutual friends, Nunzio and Santa Cannizzo, who lived two doors away from the Vassallos. During early summer, my father approached Mrs. Cannizzo and confessed his great love for Vincenza, asking her if she would bring notes from him to Vincenza. Mrs. Cannizzo proceeded to be the liaison between the two lovers, and for six months notes went back and forth.

On Christmas Eve, 1910, my father took a walk before dinner. The desire to get a glimpse of Vincenza had been tormenting him, so he headed directly for her street, hoping that she was out on her terrace. The streets were empty, as everyone was with their families celebrating Christmas Eve, but my father was still afraid of being recognized. He pulled up his coat collar to hide his face.

Just as Vincenza began to close the shutters, my father's face appeared at the window. It was the closest they had ever been to each other. They called to each other by name, and heard each other's voice for the first time. She thought that since he was a farmer, his voice would be rough. Instead, he had a gentle voice.

"Do you want to elope?" my father asked.

"Yes! Wait while I get my shawl." In a matter of seconds, my mother came out into the dimly lit street with her black shawl over her head. My father spoke to her gently, making her joyous to be with him.

The possibility of being discovered frightened my father. Acting on an impulse, he knocked on the Cannizzos' door, just down the street. When Nunzio saw them together, he immediately pulled them inside and shut the door, realizing what was going on. Meanwhile, Vincenza's mother, Cristina, discovered her daughter missing and grasped what had transpired. She ran out into the street, shouting frantically that my father had stolen her daughter from under her eye, and sent neighbors to call her sons. Shortly thereafter, her two sons came, carrying shotguns, and searched the street, but to no avail. No one imagined that the lovers were only two doors away.

About 3:00 A.M., the streets were deserted, and Mr. Cannizzo suggested that it would be a good time to go. He and his wife were worried about their involvement in the mess.

MCKENZIE'S DUKE, A SPECIAL DOG

In 1950, I learned that Bobby, my eight-year-old beagle, had an incurable illness. Bobby was an excellent hunting dog, and we had spent six happy years together. Three veterinarians agreed that I should put him to sleep. I took their advice, saying good-bye to Bobby with a big hug and tears rolling down my face.

Arriving back at the shop, I was greeted by one of my clients, Benjamin Mintz, president of Trinity Bag Company, who had come in for his daily shave. After his shave, noting my air of sadness, he asked what was wrong. I told him about Bobby, adding that I felt like I had lost my best friend. He expressed his sympathy, and then said that I should buy another dog and he would pay for it.

Another client, Jack Long, a hunter and president of a railroad company in Chicago, visited my shop whenever he was on a business trip to New York. He had told me that if I ever needed a beagle, to let him know. I called him, and within one week I received a letter from a kennel saying that Mr. Long had spoken to them and they had a dog for me.

The dog's name was McKenzie's Duke. He was two years old, fully trained, and had won two ribbons in field trials. Duke was shipped by Railway Express, and he arrived looking strong and healthy, but very shy.

Duke was a superb hunter. Even with other dogs around him, Duke, unleashed, would remain by my side. Duke even refused to hunt with my partners unless I was there. Also, he rarely hunted with other dogs; he preferred to hunt individually.

On one of our hunting trips, we saw a young doe, the size of a goat, tempting Duke to give chase. The deer would gain ground easily, stop until Duke was within fifty feet, and take off again. She did this twice and then went over the hill, with Duke in hot pursuit. Meanwhile, it was snowing heavily, making driving very dangerous. We decided to go

My father and Vincenza went out into the night, Vincenza with the black shawl covering her head and my father with his coat collar up and his head down, making their way south on Via Salanitro—the long way, so there would be less chance of meeting anyone.

The road was deserted. They went around the southern end of the Castello Santapau, up the desolate promenade, holding each other, past the many caves left by the earthquake that destroyed the castle. When they arrived at my grandfather's house, they were welcomed and embraced by him and my father's sister, Giuseppa. They did their utmost to make my mother feel welcome and comfortable.

On December 26, my parents were married. The Vassallos were invited, but they chose not to attend. My mother was promptly criticized by her family and did not receive the dowry of the size due her.

About six months later, hearing of my mother's happiness and the news that Vincenza was expecting to give birth in September, my grandmother Cristina, her sons Nunzio and Francesco, and their wives went to visit my parents, breaking the ice by announcing that her generous dowry, a property at Giurfo, would be given to her. This was a great location, a paradise in the summer, and everyone who had property there brought their families for the season. Half of the property consisted of 13,000 vines of grapes, and almond, olive, and fruit trees; the other half was planted for grain. My birth on September 27, 1911, brought greater harmony to the already favorable conditions.

My uncle Francesco and his wife, Margaret, who had no children of their own, were elated. They shared a special feeling for my mother, because she was the youngest daughter who grew up with them. My grandmother Cristina lived with them in the same house. As I grew up, they spoiled me, which was not appreciated by my parents. I reciprocated their deep-felt sentiments.

As time passed, my father became my grandmother's favorite son-in-law, just as my mother was her pride and joy. In the early part of 1913, my father became aware of opportunities in the United States, when people coming back from America after only a few years had money to buy land and houses. They told him that anyone willing to work could find work easily in the States. The idea of being able to buy their own house instead of home, and I told the caretaker about Duke's disappearance over the hill, adding that I would call him later.

The return trip took four hours instead of the usual two. I immediately called the caretaker. Duke had come back, but he wouldn't go into the house and refused to eat. He just lay in the snow where we had parked our car.

The next morning, Duke was still lying in the snow where we had parked. I immediately took a train back to Patterson, New York. When I finally arrived, there was Duke—he hadn't moved. I called him, and he ran to me, jumping all over me with happiness. At the railroad station, I bought Duke two hamburgers, which he gulped down. Arriving back at the shop, I put two Turkish towels on the floor for him to lie on.

That night, Duke had a special supper with me, and then went to his doghouse to dream about the deer that made a fool out of him. He never chased a deer again!

living in my grandfather's house (although we were most welcome) was appealing to him. He discussed the idea with my mother, making it clear that I would have to be left behind with her mother, brother, and sister-in-law, a saintly woman who treated me as her own.

2

IN the summer of 1913, my parents arrived in New York. They were met by the family of Vincenzo Tillona, who proposed that they live in their apartment at 204 Mott Street in Manhattan until they could find one of their own. The Tillonas had two children, Antoinette and Tom.

My father didn't speak English, was without a trade, and had no choice but to do manual work on the docks. My mother, an excellent seamstress, found immediate employment in a women's coat factory. Working conditions on the docks were terrible. The Irish foreman forced the workers to give him 25¢ a week under the table, or else be out of work. The foreman was the only one who spoke English. Every day, my father tied up a chunk of ice at the docks and dragged it home for the ice box, saving the trolley fare and the price of the ice. Despite all these hardships, my parents were happy. They could see their plans materializing.

But in 1914, war began between Italy and Germany. The Italian government announced that all Italian citi-

ELI COHN, THE RESULTS OF A CONCENTRATION CAMP

In the late 1940s, I put an ad in the Help Wanted section of the New York *Journal American* for a barber. Eli Cohn was one of the five barbers who answered the ad. He was about thirty-five years old, short and bald, with a round face and reddish complexion. Although he spoke little English, he was experienced, personable, eager to work, and an excellent barber. He learned our method of scalp treatments and face massages in short order.

After Eli had been with us about three months, he came in one morning and said that lately, on his way home, someone he recognized from the concentration camp was following him. He still had vivid nightmares of the German concentration camps and of seeing his mother and father killed. Sometimes, as he gave a massage, I heard a particular customer complain that he was pressing too hard on his throat with his fingers. I

zens living abroad must return to Italy immediately, to fight for their country. Italian citizens who didn't comply would be prohibited from returning to Italy at a later date. My father argued that if he went back, he would be drafted in the Italian army and would soon be sent to the front. But no amount of reasoning outweighed my mother's resolve to go back to Italy. Their plans for the future were suddenly overshadowed by war.

On my parents' arrival in Licodia Eubea, my father was inducted into military service. My mother and I went to live with my grandmother Cristina, my uncle Francesco, and his wife. Because of my father's education in the priesthood, he was immediately made a sergeant major. He was sent to the Austrian front, where he fought for two years.

Then a grenade fragment injured him above his right eye, and he ended up in a field hospital. Two days later, a combined German and Austrian advance took the doctors and nurses, hospital personnel, and wounded prisoners. The ambulatory prisoners walked for two days until they reached trains that would take them to prison camps in Frankfurt, Germany. During a train change, they were joined by other prisoners from other trains, and among them my father recognized my uncle Francesco. They embraced each other with joy, happy that they were together. After they arrived at a station near Frankfurt, there were two more days of walking. During this period, a German soldier walking the prisoners relentlessly picked on Uncle Francesco, who had always been physically frail, for not keeping up with everyone. Other prisoners, noticing this harassment, became angry and passed the word on in Italian to throw the German over the bridge they were crossing. At the center of the bridge, in an instant, he was grabbed and flung over the side. The noise of the rushing water drowned out his cries, and in the pitch black night, the act went unnoticed.

When they reached the prison camp, my father and uncle were separated. As a blessing from heaven, my father was assigned to the kitchen. Eventually, he became the supervisor and cooked only for the German officers. He won his captors over to the idea of allowing him to go in and out of the camp, particularly to buy supplies for the officers. This freedom, and his status, enabled him to get extra food to his starving comrades.

am certain that client's features reminded Eli of a German capo.

Eli was now doing very well in the shop. Many clients made appointments with him, especially Jewish clients. One morning, he didn't come to work. He didn't call, and I couldn't call him, as he had no phone. He suddenly appeared three days later, very dirty looking, with a three-day beard. His eyes were bloodshot. He looked exhausted and troubled. I asked what happened. He said that when he left the shop Monday night, he recognized a German from the concentration camp waiting for him. The man followed Eli, who changed subways three times, ending at Pennsylvania Station where he took a train to Washington. The man followed Eli there for two days, until Eli finally eluded him. He came back to New York this morning.

I said, "Eli, am I your friend? Do you trust me?" He said yes. I suggested that he let me take him to Bellevue Hospital, but he insisted that he wasn't crazy. I assured him

I knew he wasn't crazy, but if he were admitted there, he could get some rest and would be safe. When he was released, he could come back to work. He agreed.

I went to get my jacket, and when I returned, Eli was gone. Three months later, I received a letter from his brother in Israel telling me that Eli had flung himself in front of a train in Boston, the day after I almost saved his life.

After two long years in the prison camp, the armistice was signed on November 11, 1918. My father was released from military duty and prison camp. My uncle had gotten home before him, and I looked upon him as a paternal figure. I was now seven years old and didn't accept my father as my real father. Uncle Francesco had been home longer, giving me love and attention. Once, when my father tried to reprimand me, I told my mother to throw him out of the house. But slowly, with patience and know-how, he won me over.

Despite his large landholdings, my father decided against working as a farmer. Instead, he opened a modern café. He found a perfect location on Corso Umberto I, the main street. It consisted of an apartment in the back with a balcony overlooking the countryside and the store in front. It was named the Café Aurora. My father went to Catania to take a course in running a café so he would have an edge over the three other cafés in town. In the city, after completing the course, he bought machinery to bottle the favorite soft drink there called Cazzosa. It came in twelve-ounce bottles with a bulge in the middle of the neck where a glass ball floated. The machine, after filling the bottle, brought the ball to the lip of the bottle and sealed it with compression. To open, you pushed the ball with your thumb, and it fell down to the bulge of the neck. He also invested in a machine to make gelati and spumoni.

My job was to serve the tables on the sidewalk and

also deliver cases of Cazzosa to other cafés in town, because it was cheaper than having them delivered from Catania. Café Aurora immediately became the busiest one in town. The other cafés were passed down from generation to generation, the heirs making no improvements. We attracted the biggest and best clientele, even though we charged higher prices. My father became very well liked and respected in the town.

On religious holidays, platforms were built in the piazza in front of the municipal building for concerts by our band and a band from a nearby town. They alternated and were very competitive. People brought chairs for their families and tied them together with the family name on them.

On special holidays, there was horse racing. The horses and their jockeys came from local towns to compete for generous purses in six races. The horsemen made their entrance into the town as the band played a march. The horses and their jockeys in colorful silks were followed by a crowd of men and children. The race was the length of the main street, starting at the piazza in front of the Church Madrici and ending at the entrance to the town, about a half mile away. These holidays were always great events. There were vendors from out of town with carts selling all kinds of food to eat, plus many games of skill for both children and grown-ups. This meant extra business for our café, which was on the main street about two hundred and fifty feet from the band platform. We were kept busy and prosperous. But around October of 1919, this came to a sudden end.

The Italian government announced that men who had come from the United States to fight for their country were entitled to return to the United States

R. FLEISCHMANN, PRESIDENT OF *THE NEW YORKER* IN THE 1950S

The first time Mr. Fleischmann came into our shop, I introduced him to our barber Jack Livigni. Jack shaved with the utmost care; it was his nature to work slowly but efficiently. Mr. Fleischmann was a top figure in the field of magazine publishing, and I hoped to make a client of him.

When Jack was through, Mr. Fleischmann thanked him for a wonderful shave and gave him a generous tip. Then, while he was paying his check, he said that he wanted to make a standing appointment with Jack for 10 A.M. Monday through Friday. He added that he went to his regular barber every Saturday for a haircut.

From that day on, when the clock struck ten, you would see Mr. Fleischmann's right foot enter the door to the barbershop. He invariably looked up at the clock on the wall facing him. My partner, Angelo, and I kept an eye on Jack, to make sure he was ready. Mr.

free. This ended the Café Aurora. My father felt that he would earn more money, more rapidly, if he returned to New York City. This time I would go, too.

So in December 1920, we sailed from Naples on the S.S. *Orizabba*. The ship had two decks with bunk beds, one for women and one for men. The children were given milk every day, and many times I was sent by childless couples to get them milk. The sea was very rough during the voyage. Most adults got seasick and took to their bunks. They couldn't eat. But for the children it was a ball. We weren't affected.

After twenty-one days, we landed in Philadelphia due to ice in New York Harbor. We were herded like cattle into trains bound for New York City. When we arrived in New York, we were met by a good friend of my father, Paolo DiMartino. Paolo had a wife and a three-year-old daughter, but he offered to share his three-room apartment at 125 Mott Street on the corner of Hester Street with us until we could find an apartment of our own. The DiMartinos gave the bedroom to my parents, moving their bed into the living room where their daughter had her cot. I slept in the kitchen on another cot that was opened just at night.

Mr. DiMartino took my father to the Uneeda Biscuit Company, where he got a job, and my mother was helped by another friend to get a job at a women's coat factory. I went to a public school on the corner of Hester and Baxter Streets. Frightened and lonely, I slept in my parents' bed before they came home, eating with the DiMartinos. My parents always worked overtime, usually getting home as late as 11:00 P.M. They put me on my cot when they went to bed.

In school, because of my lack of English, I was put with six-year-olds even though I was nine years old. Not being able to communicate made me very unhappy. I had had three years of school in Licodia Eubea, but it did no good here. Children made fun of my English, often calling me a wop. I got very angry and tackled them Sicilian-style, throwing them down on the ground and punching them.

As time passed, I made friends with other immigrant boys who were in the same predicament but had been in New York longer. They offered to help me if I would help them in other ways. I joined them in fights with boys who tormented them because of

Fleischmann had a reputation of being difficult. We wanted to avoid confrontations with him.

One day, Angelo was not in, and I was busy giving a shampoo to a client. Then, out of the corner of my eye, I saw Mr. Fleischmann enter the shop. According to my timetable, Jack should have been ready five minutes ago. But when I looked at Jack, I saw that he had just begun a facial massage that would take twenty minutes.

I decided that this time I wouldn't tell Mr. Fleischmann a white lie, as Angelo and I had done many times before, making Mr. Fleischmann red in the face with anger. I couldn't tell him that Jack would be busy for twenty minutes. So I went back to my client and said nothing, letting Jack face the consequences himself.

After a few minutes, Mr. Fleischmann was fidgety. Time was clicking on. He got angrier and angrier but didn't say a word. Jack called him when he finished, and Mr. Fleischmann walked slowly, looking fiercely at Jack. As Jack started preparing him for the shave, Mr. Fleischmann gave him hell in a low tone that sounded like rolling thunder. Jack apologized in a very low voice, hardly audible. Suddenly, Mr. Fleischmann yelled, "Balls!" Jack regained his composure and proceeded to shave Mr. Fleischmann without a word being said.

When the shave was finished, Mr. Fleischman gave Jack his usual tip, but without the usual thank you, then came toward me to pay for the shave. Before he said anything, I said, "Mr. Fleischmann, I would like to suggest another barber." He said, "I would like that."

their lack of English. I didn't take guff from any boy, and I was ready to defend myself at all times. From then on, fights became less frequent.

The vast majority of immigrant children where I went to school were from Sicily. I made friends mostly with them. My English was improving, but I learned it only in school, not much on the streets. After school, I worked with tailors who spoke only Italian, took violin lessons, and then studied my lessons at home where my parents never spoke English.

After two years I spoke English as well as any of the other boys. After my first two years of school, there wasn't a year that I didn't skip a class, until seventh grade. When I wasn't skipped to eighth grade, I resolved to go to summer school. I was finally promoted.

One year after my father began working at Uneeda, Cesere, a boyhood friend of my father, offered to teach him to be a presser in a women's coat factory. This was a big break, which meant that my father would be earning more than twice as much in salary.

Soon we were able to leave the DiMartinos and move into our own four-room apartment at 204 Mott Street. (This was the building my parents had lived in during their first stay in New York.) I was transferred to P.S. 21, across the street, on the corner of Spring Street. School now was more interesting to me, since I spoke English well enough to get involved in school activities. I joined the orchestra, glee club, and the baseball and track teams. I had no more problems as an immigrant boy unable to speak English.

In our new apartment, we had the luxury of a private toilet. At 125 Mott Street, there was only one toilet, in the hallway, for the use of the three or four apartments on the floor. We felt lucky having four rooms all to ourselves. The building was reasonably modern and had been well kept. I remember spending nights on our fire escape during the summer heat. Since none of our apartments had showers, once a week we went to a nearby bathhouse. We brought our own soap and towels, and paid a nickel for the shower.

My parents worked as usual, six days a week. Often they also worked on Sundays until noon. I kept busy with school and my violin lessons. Before school in the morning, I went to the subway exit on Kenmare Street in the Bowery, taking cigar bands and newspapers that people discarded. I sold the newspapers by the pound to pushcart vendors on Elizabeth Street. Finally I accumulated enough cigar bands to get a baseball glove and ball. I had my friends hold them for me, because my parents would punish me if they discovered them in the house. I was supposed to study, not waste my time playing ball.

My mother was exceptional with a needle, always being assigned to make samples of the women's coats for the factory where she worked. Eventually, my father got a job at the same factory as a presser on the pressing machines. They both were very cooperative with each other, working side by side toward their goal. They were idolized by friends and co-workers, who labeled them "Romeo and Juliet."

Whatever money my mother's farm and vineyards

back in Sicily made, my uncle Francesco put in the bank for my parents. He had as much interest in their achieving their goal as they did; he wanted them to save enough money to come back home. My mother always made more money than my father. By now she was coming home with more than $100 weekly. In Sicily, our income had been just enough to get by.

By 1926, my parents had saved enough money to buy themselves a home in Licodia Eubea. Doctor Mario Vassallo was my mother's first cousin, so they knew that the apartment at the Palazzo Vassallo was empty. He was very difficult to get along with, but since he had shown great respect for my father and mother, often coming to the Café Aurora, my father wrote to him, asking if he would consider selling them the apartment. Dr. Vassallo was elated by the idea.

In June 1927, when I was fifteen years old, I graduated from elementary school and wanted to go to high school and then to college. My grades were excellent, especially in mathematics, and my teachers told my parents that I was a very promising student. But my parents were convinced that taking me back to Sicily would be best for all of us.

Most Italian families didn't want to stay in the United States, because life was very difficult for them. Not knowing the language, they felt like fish out of water. Other than making money, there was no reason for them to stay here. They were much happier back home. I had no objection to going back to Sicily. I was convinced that a better life awaited me there.

Back in Licodia Eubea, my parents immediately hired a private tutor to prepare me for the examinations necessary to enter the *liceo*, a high school that was like a boarding school. My parents intended to leave me there and go back to New York for a further eight years, by which time I would have finished college.

After my years in New York speaking English, I now found Italian difficult, especially because my classmates were more advanced. After two months I told my parents that school was too difficult for me and I couldn't go on. If they wanted me to study, I would be happy to study in New York City, where I had no difficulty. They were keenly disappointed that I couldn't go on at the *liceo*, and they tried very hard to change my mind.

Studying in New York City was definitely out. They suggested that I decide on a trade. We would go back to New York City, work together for a few more years, buy some land, and then return together. Not knowing what trade to choose, I left it to my parents to decide. They proposed barbering, which was easy to learn, so that I could quickly start earning money. The next day, my father took me to a master barber, Ferdinando Vassallo (he was related to my mother). He agreed to teach me barbering and told me to report to work the following day.

During our six-month stay in Sicily, my parents modernized the apart-

SCALP TREATMENT SHAMPOO

1. Put steamed towel over the head.
2. Put therapeutic red lamp on stand over head and hot towel.
3. Take off hot towel and leave lamp.
4. Have warm lotion for the individual's scalp (kept warm in compartment over sterilizer).
5. Put warm lotion for dry, normal, or oily hair on scalp.
6. Massage scalp slowly with vibrator for three full minutes.
7. Apply shampoo.
8. Rub shampoo in slowly, throwing excessive foam into sink, for about one minute.
9. Bring client to sink and rinse twice.
10. Finish off with hair dressing suggested by barber, or use client's choice.

ment, adding four rooms above the two back rooms and a large terrace that offered vast views on all sides. There was also a water tank with a pump that brought water up from the cistern below. Dr. Vassallo gave us the right to use the cistern that had rainwater. We had a large clay jug for drinking water that we got daily from the fountain half a block away, where it was kept cool.

3

IN January of 1928, after I had had three months of basic barbering, we returned to New York City. I registered at the Manhattan Barber School, located in the Bowery, where I actually practiced since I already knew the basics. I was at the school for four weeks. For the first two weeks, I was assigned to the free service section. For the next two weeks I cut hair in the advanced department, charging 5¢ for a shave and 10¢ for a haircut.

My father introduced me to a friend of his, Sebastian Bonvicino, who owned a barber shop on the Bowery between Hester and Canal Streets. The shop was in a basement under a restaurant and employed eight barbers. It was patronized by the same people who came to the barber school. Many were so drunk that they fell down on the stairs. We would pick them up and put them in the barber chair. Oddly, they never seemed to get hurt. Some of them obviously didn't belong there, but the breaks of life had brought them to the bottom. From these customers we always requested payment in advance: 10¢ for a shave and 20¢ for a haircut. Often they tipped more than the basic service charges. They probably understood what we were putting up with and a few even apologized for their condition. Our hours were 8:00 A.M. to 8:00 P.M., and until 10:00 P.M. on Saturdays. My salary was $6 a week.

After two months at Mr. Bonvicino's barbershop, my father asked another friend, Pietro DiGrazia, if he could use an apprentice at his barbershop on Eldridge Street. Mr. DiGrazia said he could, and I went to work the following Monday. Thankfully there were no drunkards. Mr. DiGrazia was very good to me and gave me every opportunity to learn to be a better barber.

After a couple of months, as winter was approaching, Mr. DiGrazia said that in cold weather I would have to arrive at 7:00 A.M. to stoke the stove with coal so that the shop would be warm when it opened at 8 o'clock. I didn't relish the job. I bought the *Journal American*, in which barbershop owners advertised for barbers. One day, I found an advertisement for a barber on West Thirty-seventh Street. I asked Mr. DiGrazia for a couple of hours off to apply for a better job (he was paying me $10 a week). He said, "Sure," and wished me luck.

At 9:00 A.M. the next morning, I arrived at the barbershop on Thirty-seventh Street. The owner, a Greek immigrant named Charlie Demitros, was sorry to say that the position had been filled at 8:00 A.M. I vowed to arrive early next time I applied for a job. As I was about to go, Charlie asked me for my home address, in case he wasn't pleased with the barber he'd hired. I liked the shop. It was clean and orderly, with four chairs and four barbers. There were two doors to the shop, one on the street and the other from the lobby of the building. I was fascinated to see six canaries, each in an individual cage, hanging in the shop, singing and making it cheerful. I left my name and address but told him that I couldn't work six days a week, because I needed a half day for my violin lessons. Suddenly Charlie announced that I was hired. He said, "I own a violin. I want you to teach me to play it. I'll pay you for the full six days in return." I was thrilled.

I began work the following Monday. The first week, I earned a $10 commission in addition to my basic $20 salary, plus $5 in tips. The proper salary was $20 weekly, plus 50 percent above $35 gross taken on the chair, giving the owner a profit of $15 plus 50 percent above the $35 gross. Starting the second week, Charlie made me the manager of the shop, raising my salary to $25. This was a big jump from the $10 I earned at Mr. DiGrazia's shop.

Charlie was often away from the shop. He painted murals in restaurants and was busy buying and selling canaries. But he was usually in the shop on Saturday, the busiest day of the week. Charlie was a fifty-year-old bachelor who would obviously never learn to play the violin. But he gave it all he had at his weekly lessons. He loved to hear me play his violin, and I loved to play it. It was supposedly signed by Stradivarius, but so were many copies. You could never be sure. But to this day, I believe it was an original.

I worked for Charlie for about six months, finally leaving him for what I thought was a better job. I made four attempts to find a better job and failed each time. But if I was fired on Saturday, I got a job the following Monday in another shop. I remember counting the different places I worked the first eighteen

THOMAS MCLOUD, PRESIDENT OF THE FIRST STERN'S DEPARTMENT STORE

Thomas McLoud was six foot three, weighed 230 pounds, and had steel gray eyes that looked right through you. He was of Scottish descent, about fifty years old, and lived in Bayshore, Long Island. One day, after I finished his daily shave, he asked me why I shaved him in half the time that other barbers did. I said, "As you are an unusually good tipper, other barbers are extra careful, using short strokes with their razor, whereas I use long strokes on everyone, including you. Also, you may intimidate them with your stern look. I'm never intimidated by any client, because I can always replace him, even you."

When I was through with him, he said, "Pat, put your coat on and come with me." I followed him to the men's department in his store. He then called one of the salesmen, telling him to fit me with a suit and a coat and charge it to

months, from January 1928 to July 1929. There were seventeen. Each time I was let go, Charlie always took me back.

During this period I also went to Speciale's Barber Agency. They sent me to a shop on University Place and Twelfth Street. When I arrived at the shop the owner said, "I don't want a boy. I want a man with experience. Go back and tell Mr. Speciale what I said." Back at the agency, Mr. Speciale was angry. He put on his hat and coat and said, "Come with me." At the barbershop (which was only a short distance from the agency), he gave hell to the boss, asking if he had ever disappointed him before. He said he knew what he was doing and told the boss to try me.

The boss gave me a barber jacket and assigned a chair to me. Soon a client came in, and I proceeded to cut his hair, with the owner watching my every move. Another client came in and he had him wait for me, and then another. When I was through with my third client, it was now almost noon. I went to the boss and asked him if he liked my work. He said, "Very good. I guess you want to go to lunch now?" I said, "No. Pay me for the three haircuts I did. I won't work for you because you wouldn't at least give me a trial when I applied for the job this morning, instead of humiliating me." He apologized and offered me $2 more a week if I would stay. I refused. After he paid me, I went to Mr. Speciale and explained what had transpired. He said, "Good. He deserved it."

One day I applied for a job in a shop on East Eighteenth Street, owned by Rocco Quarato. Rocco was from Altamura in the province of Bari. He asked me to come back that evening to try me out on a haircut and a shave. That evening, Rocco had a model with very difficult hair and a tough beard to test me. By this time I was confident of my work and had no problem getting the job. The job paid $20 per week plus commission and tips. The prices here were higher than at Charlie's. The shop had excellent trade in the Gramercy Park area, including judges and politicians from nearby Tammany Hall.

To my amazement, the first afternoon I worked there, Rocco took out a mandolin and started playing. When I told him that I played the violin, he told me to bring my violin the next day and he would bring his guitar. At 3:30 the next afternoon we gave our first concert. He played very well and so did I, even though I had stopped taking lessons months before.

him. From that day forward, we became good friends.

On special events and holidays, there were parties for the employees of Stern's. The parties usually ended at about 2:00 A.M. Mr. McLoud would tell everyone that he was driving home to Bayshore, and would be back at 9:30 A.M. Instead, he had a room reserved at the Biltmore Hotel a block away. The next morning he would be awakened at 8 o'clock and be on time for his 8:30 appointment with me. I would shave him and give him a revitalizing face and body massage, and then he would have a good breakfast at the restaurant next door and be in the store at 9:30 sharp, looking terrific, while all the others dragged themselves in late, looking haggard. He made sure that he was seen by everyone. Then he disappeared and returned to the Biltmore to go to bed. He returned to the store at 4:30. I never revealed his secret to his workers.

WINSTON CHURCHILL

About 1939, Winston Churchill was barnstorming throughout the United States, trying to sell Americans the idea that in the event of a war with Nazi Germany, we belonged on the side of Great Britain. His lecture manager, Harold Peet, had been a client of mine since 1935. His office was just a block from my first barbershop. Early one afternoon, Mr. Peet called to ask if I had time to trim Mr. Churchill's hair. I told Mr. Peet to bring Mr. Churchill in twenty minutes.

Mr. Churchill was charming. As I worked on him, I enjoyed his British accent as he spoke to Mr. Peet, who sat on a stool next to the chair. At times, I could not see to cut his hair, due to the cloud of smoke spiraling up from his Havana cigar. It had a great aroma. When I finished, he told me how pleased he was with the trim and the wonderful service, and gave me $5, promising to see me again when he returned to New York on his next tour. Less than a year later, he was made prime minister.

Our concert became a daily event. People passing by would stop to listen; a few even came into the shop. As we played, the other two barbers were busy, and clients who wanted Rocco or me would wait until 4:30, the end of our concert. In no time at all, I was making $25 to $30 in commission and another $25 or $30 in tips, plus my $20 basic salary. Within six months, I had built a large following.

One day, as we finished a concert, a man came into the shop clapping his hands, saying, "Bravo, bravo." He said, "How would you like to play on the radio for a *paesano* of yours?" We asked who the *paesano* was. He said, "Fiorello LaGuardia. He is running for mayor of New York City." The man was in charge of a Spanish program recommending LaGuardia for mayor, and he asked us if we would play some Spanish music for the half-hour program. We said we would be happy to, adding that we would bring two friends to play guitar and bass. We practiced for two evenings and were ready with more Spanish songs than the program could ever use. (Our music did not help Mr. LaGuardia get elected, though he made it on his next try.)

When we finished playing, a gentleman complimented us and introduced himself as the owner of a drugstore a few blocks from our shop. He begged us to come to his house to play at his daughter's sweet-sixteen party. He wanted to surprise her with our quartet. We were very happy to play, but Rocco had promised his wife that he would come home an hour after the program ended. So we agreed to play for only an hour. When we got to the party, we quickly got into the swing, eating, drinking, and playing. We played on without looking at the time. The next thing we knew it was 4:00 A.M.

Rocco arrived home at 5:00 A.M. When he tried to open the door, he found it bolted. He rang the doorbell, but his wife refused to open it. Rocco headed for his brother-in-law Paul's house, a couple of blocks away. It took Paul a full week to persuade Rocco's wife to forgive him. Yet he was not absolved until he promised in front of the whole family that it would never happen again.

About a month later, the radio station called to tell us that olive oil, cheese, and macaroni companies all wanted to hire our quartet for radio advertising. Rocco's wife wouldn't give him permission, and we had to decline.

That was the price Rocco paid for marrying for money. He had been working for Paul, when Paul confessed that he had a sister-in-law living with him and his wife. She worked as a seamstress in a clothing factory, making good money. She had $1,000 in the bank and wanted to get married. Immediately, Rocco began to think seriously about her and her $1,000. He soon told Paul he was interested in her, and within three months they were married. A few months later, Rocco bought his barbershop—for $1,000. He was happy to

WALTER WEISS, LAWYER AND WRITER OF LAWTEX BOOKS

Walter Weiss was a distinguished-looking gentleman. He was in his mideighties, with beautiful white wavy hair and a full mustache. He always smiled and was soft-spoken.

Mr. Weiss was retired, and his chauffeur drove him to the shop every four weeks for a haircut and hot olive oil shampoo. On entering the shop, following his warm greeting to us, he went to the magazine table and picked up the latest *Playboy* and *Penthouse*. He then sat down in the barber chair, with the magazines on his lap. When Angelo or I finished, he paid his check and tipped. He then sat in one of the four waiting chairs and slowly looked through the magazines, holding them about six inches from his nose. (He could see best at a short distance without glasses.) The magazine reading took about forty-five minutes. His chauffeur waited patiently in the lobby.

have realized his dream of owning his own barbershop but never guessed that Lucretia, his wife, would eventually become the boss. It was, after all, her money that paid for it.

I discovered that she was the boss about a year later. One Saturday evening, Rocco told me that his wife said I was making too much money for a young man only nineteen years old. She wanted to cut my weekly base salary from $20 to $18. I refused to accept the cut, and I quit. The following Monday morning, I went back to Speciale's Barber Agency. Mr. Speciale didn't blame me for quitting, yet was sorry to tell me that I wouldn't make half as much on any job he could give me. Then he offered me a job on Lafayette street, south of Canal Street, that paid $20 a week plus commission, just like Rocco's. The first week, I made only $3 commission and $10 in tips, compared to $25 and $30 commission and $25 to $30 in tips at Rocco's.

The following week, I asked the boss for Tuesday morning off, as I had an errand to do. That morning, I went to visit the tailor next door to Rocco's barbershop. Someone told Rocco that I was in the tailor shop, and immediately Rocco came in, greeting me heartily. (This had been my plan.)

Rocco asked me if I was working, and I said, "Yes, and not only do I get the same salary, but I have every Tuesday morning off." Rocco explained that cutting my pay had been his wife's idea, and he offered me my job back. I accepted, if he would give me a $2-a-week raise in my basic salary to $22, or give me a morning off as they did in my new job. He said okay, as long as it was between us. His wife must never know that my pay was more than $18. Rocco offered to give me the $4 difference himself. We shook hands.

That afternoon, I explained my situation to my employer, telling him what I was going to do. He said, "I understand. I don't blame you. I knew you were too good to be true." He called the barber agency, and Mr. Speciale assured him that he would have another good barber for him next morning. I went back to Rocco's the next morning. Rocco and my clients were very happy. Of course, I was, too!

Around this time, I started noticing Connie DiMartino, the daughter of my parents' friend John DiMartino. John also came from Licodia Eubea, and his wife, Catherine, came from Musilmeri, in the province of Palermo.

One day after his usual appointment, he called Angelo and me aside and told us that he was guilty of undertipping us for years with only 25¢. "Starting today," he announced, "I will begin making up for it." He gave Angelo a $20 tip. We figured that because of his advanced age, he believed he didn't have much time to make it up. He was such a fine gentleman that we never held the 25¢ tip against him. Thereafter, if our *Playboy* and *Penthouse* magazines were the current issues, he tipped $20. If they were older, he tipped $15.

Shortly after this, Mr. Weiss became ill. After four months, I received a call from Mrs. Weiss asking if I could come to their apartment to give Mr. Weiss a haircut and shave. Of course, I accepted. I found him looking like Santa Claus, with four months' pure white hair and full beard. He chased his wife and nurse out of the room, and the first thing he wanted to know was if I had brought the magazines. I had not, but I promised the next time I would not forget them. I asked him, however, why he did not subscribe to them. He said, "My wife won't let me."

When I was finished, Mrs. Weiss came in with a checkbook and asked how much to make out the check for. Mr. Weiss replied, "Make it for seventy-five dollars," winking at me.

Mr. Weiss died about two months later, without the pleasure of looking through *Playboy* or *Penthouse* again. They probably helped keep him alive. At least, they made him happy.

The DiMartinos lived in Riverdale, in a mansion on nearly an acre of land, with fruit trees and a big iron gate at the entrance of the property. John and Catherine had seven children, five girls and two boys, of whom Connie was the oldest. Our families celebrated holidays together, either in Riverdale or at our apartment. I noticed Connie being very attentive to me, and I became attracted to her as well. (What I didn't know was that Connie had her eyes on me long before I noticed. Later on she confessed that she had decided that I would be her man when she was about twelve, and she never dated anyone but me.)

As time went on, I started to notice her kindness, gentleness, and willingness to help others. She was very much a lady. I asked her to come to see me at the shop. To do that, she had to tell a small lie to her father, saying that she was going to the movies. Then she would take a trolley and then the subway down to Eighteenth Street. I would take her to dinner, along with an ice cream soda, and take the subway with her and watch her board the trolley home. Then I took the subway to my home, which now was in Brooklyn. It took me two hours.

As we got to know each other, I began taking Connie to the movies. One night, after about ten minutes, I put my arm around her shoulder. As I did that, she moved to the next seat. I moved over as well and again attempted to put my arm around her. My arm never made it; she moved again. I followed, moving to the next seat. This happened four times. Then I got angry, telling her that if she moved one more time, I would go home and never go to the movies with her again. She didn't budge. It went this way for almost two years.

In the summer of 1932, my parents told me that the time had arrived to return to Licodia Eubea permanently. We already owned properties that produced wheat, grapes, olives, almonds, and all kinds of fruits. They were to be left as they were. My father and I planned an additional venture.

There were three or four men who came daily from Catania by train and stagecoach to our town, two hours each way. Each had a very large basket, and they went from house to house buying extra eggs from housewives who raised chickens behind their homes. Each evening the men went back home to sell their baskets full of eggs, making enough money to support their families and to pay for their transportation. Our idea was to live in town and to encourage families living in the country to raise chickens for extra income. We would have a truck and visit the farms daily, supervising the work and bringing eggs and chickens to the city as often as necessary. Nothing like that existed. Also, it would be a great opportunity for the farmers.

When my parents told me that my Uncle Francesco had girls from fine families with big dowries for me to pick from, I knew it was time to tell them about Connie. I said that we were very serious about each other and I intended to ask Connie to marry me and come back to Licodia Eubea with us. My mother and father were delighted. I called Connie and fixed a time to see her the next day.

We met at a restaurant near the shop, and I confessed that I was in love with her. I asked if she would marry me and move back to Sicily. She immediately said yes.

As was Sicilian custom, my parents visited Connie's father. They asked for Connie's hand in marriage to me. They also explained their plans. Of course, John was sad to lose his oldest daughter, but he knew that she would have a good life with us.

We planned for a September engagement party at Connie's house, setting December 11 as our wedding date. The party was an elaborate affair in the large, dome-ceilinged living room with doors to the patio and the garden. Later, we made preparations for our wedding. We expected a large turnout of both families and their many friends.

Our wedding day was dismal and cold, with freezing rain. It was tricky to walk because the ground was a sheet of ice. But that didn't stop nearly one thousand people from coming to the reception. Connie had to be carried to the car to go to St. Margherite's Church in Riverdale. Father Doyle, who later became a monsignor, performed the ceremony.

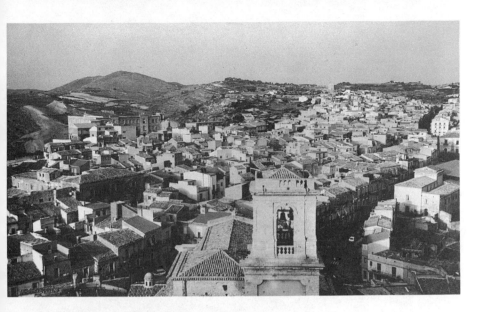

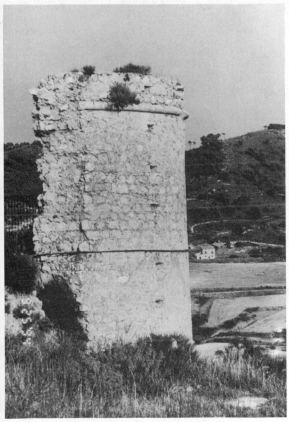

Top: Panorama of Licodia Eubea from the grounds of Santapao Castle. Large dark building at left center is Palazzo Vassallo.

Left: The last standing turret of Santapao Castle.

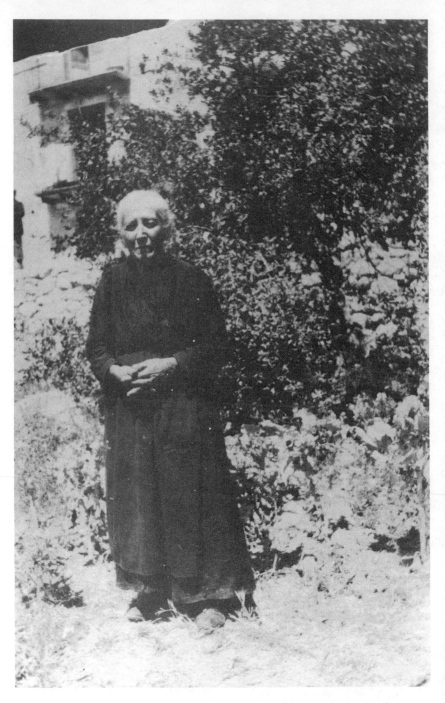

My grandmother Christina.

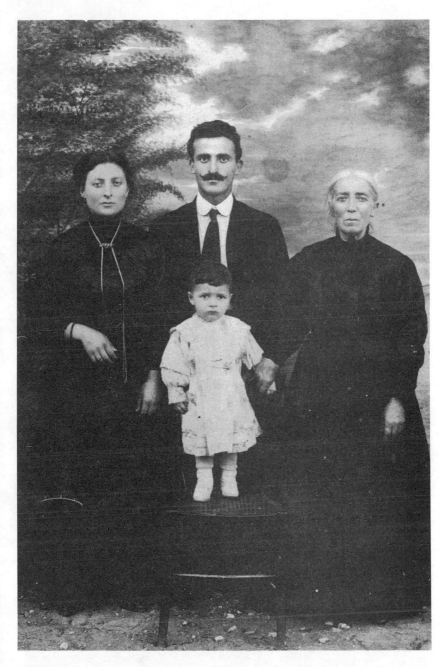

My family with me in 1913, before my parents came to New York City for the first time. From left to right: my mother, father, and grandmother Christina.

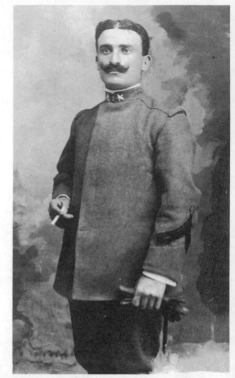

Right: My father, Francesco Spagnuolo, at the Austrian front in World War I in 1915.

Below: My father, at left, drinking wine with other soldiers in 1915.

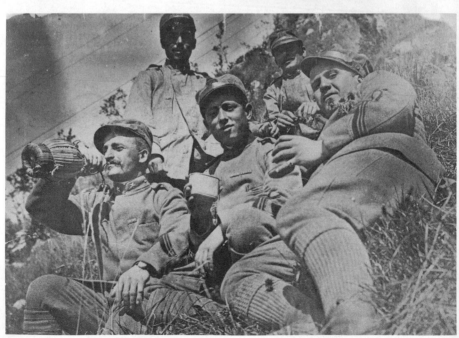

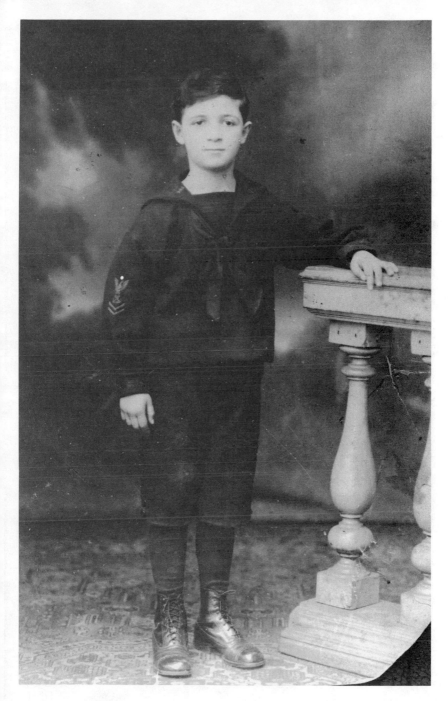

Here I am at eleven years old.

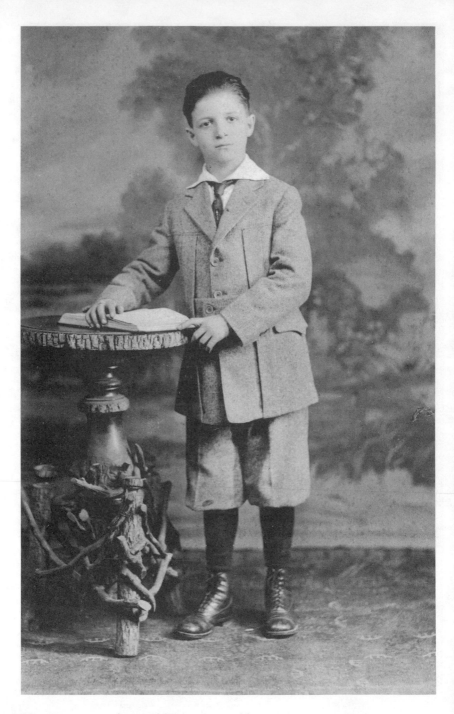

Here I am at twelve or thirteen years old.

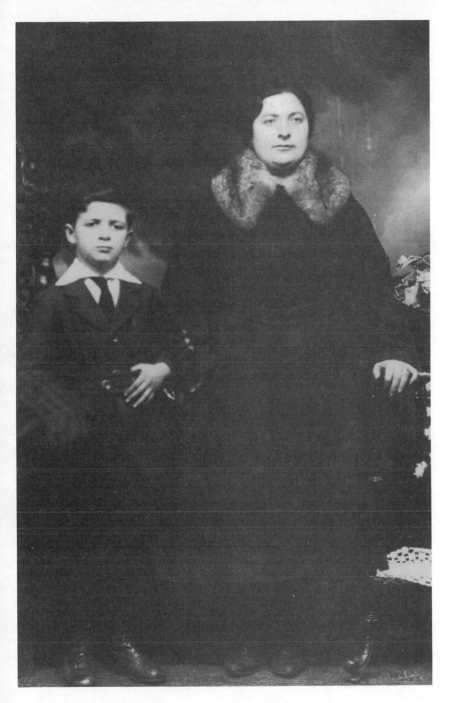

My mother, Vincenza, with me in 1923 in New York City.

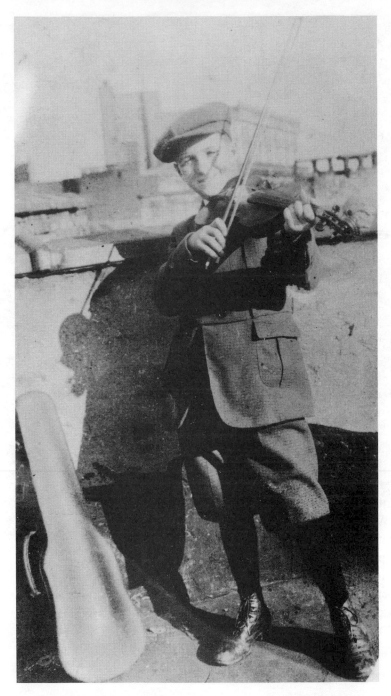

I am fourteen years old, playing a tune on the roof of 204 Mott Street in New York City.

4

WE sailed for Sicily on the *Saturnia* on March 4, 1933. That morning we were to pick up $1,000 at my bank for spending money. Imagine our dilemma to find that the bank was closed until further notice, by order of President Franklin D. Roosevelt. Fortunately, many friends came to see us off, and they gave us all the money they had on them.

The voyage was wonderful. Thanks to our best man, Vincent Palmer, who ran a travel agency, we were in first-class cabins with twin beds and a private bath. The ship toured the Azores, Lisbon, Gibraltar, and Cannes before docking at Palermo.

When the *Saturnia* arrived in Palermo, many rowboats filled with shouting people gathered around the ship. Suddenly we heard, "Spagnuolo! Spagnuolo!" We yelled back, "Vassallo! Vassallo!" My uncle Francesco, upon hearing us call back, started waving his arms. Two hours later, we were embracing each other. Connie and Uncle Francesco were delighted to meet each other, but conversation was difficult since Connie

MILK DELIVERY TO YOUR DOOR—BY GOAT!

At 7:30 every morning, we heard the bells from about twenty goats coming up our street. Connie would go to the balcony and watch them approach our home. When the goatherd walking behind them gave the lead goat a command to stop, the others also stopped. Our goat knew our house after about a week, and would leave the pack and make its way up about thirty steps to our door with the goatherd following. Connie would be waiting with a pitcher for the goatherd to fill with milk from the goat. When the goatherd finished milking, the goat would run down the stairs, happy to be rid of the weight of the milk.

The typical arrangement for this service was that you would buy the goat and give it to the goatherd to take care of on a fifty-fifty basis. Goats give milk twice daily. The goatherd would bring you milk every morning with your goat. He kept the evening milk, from which he made

couldn't speak Italian. They reached each other through their smiles and gestures.

In six hours we arrived at Licodia Eubea. It was nightfall, and Connie looked around, confused and puzzled about what she had gotten herself into. Entering Uncle Francesco's house, we were greeted and embraced by my Grandmother Cristina and my Aunt Margaret and other relatives. Everyone made a fuss over the American girl. They talked to her, but she was at a loss, not being able to express herself, just saying *"grazie."* That's all the Italian she knew.

Connie was disappointed by my uncle's house because it was so small. It had three rooms and a terrace overlooking the countryside. Two of the rooms were used as bedrooms, and the other large room was used as a kitchen, dining, and living room. There were two rooms below the first floor, and below that was the stable. Because the stable was at street level at the back of the house, and the main floor of the house was also at street level, but a flight higher, after dark the whole apartment seemed gloomy. Aunt Margaret, an unusually kind person, took Connie by the hand and guided her from room to room, then down the dingy stairway to the two mezzanine rooms. They were dark with no windows, used for supplies and clothes. I realized just in time that Aunt Margaret was about to take Connie down another flight to the stables and the roosting chickens. Connie was very relieved when I told Aunt Margaret not to take her down there, because there would be other times. Her heart was black, obviously thinking, Where has Pat taken me? The furniture was very old. People, even people of means, lived the same way they always had. Only immigrants to America who returned to Licodia Eubea lived a more contemporary way of life, and they were often criticized by the townspeople for their lifestyle.

cheese. When the goat gave birth to one offspring, you could take it after the milk feeding period and give the goatherd half of the going price. If you chose not to take it, the goatherd gave you the equivalent price in cheese. In the case of two offspring, you and the goatherd got one each. The goatherd would supply you with your morning milk from one of his own goats until the weaning period.

This service ended in Licodia Eubea in the spring of 1935, when Benito Mussolini declared war on Ethiopia.

My grandmother and Aunt Margaret and relatives, some of them from Connie's father's family, had prepared all kinds of delicious food and goodies for the festivities. When we finished eating, I announced that Connie had been pregnant for two months. It was a joyous occasion, with toasts of wine made from our grapes at Shili Sotto.

After the meal, we walked to our house. I kept reassuring Connie about our beautiful home, but her smile was forced. She didn't believe me. But when we arrived, Connie was suddenly radiant. She was in awe of the large entrance with the Vassallo family crest above the door. A truck could drive through it. As we entered to the left, there were four steps to a platform and to the right sixteen steps to another platform and then left again another four steps to our apartment. As we entered, I turned on the electric lights. She went from room to room, amazed at their size. Our bedroom was twenty-seven feet square with a large door to a balcony on Via Mugnos with a view of the Castello Santapao and the church. The ceilings of cathedral height were made of pumice, with sculpture on each corner where it met the wall. The floors were terrazzo tiles with beautiful designs. Our closet was a walk-in, five feet by twenty feet. Now Connie apologized for having doubted me, saying that everything I had told her was true and much more beautiful than she had dreamed.

That summer of 1933, we went to my parents' property, the land given as a dowry to my mother by her widowed mother. The location was well known for its vineyards and fruit trees. On half of our property, there were 13,000 grapevines, almond trees, olive trees, fruit trees, and cactus plants with prickly pears. On the remainder were grown grain and fava beans, in alternating years for a better crop.

On summer evenings it was a ritual to take long walks to visit friends, tasting each other's homemade food and cordials. There was always someone who played the guitar or the mandolin, or who sang. The sky in the evening was lovely, clear and bright with stars.

Many evenings, I was asked to play my violin for young men wanting to serenade their girlfriends. Once, when we were playing music under a balcony, the father of the girl came out, telling us off in no uncertain terms. The young man who was singing his heart out said that the girl loved him, in spite of her father. We continued playing and within five minutes, he appeared again on the balcony, this time with a white porcelain pot in his hand. We recognized it as a chamber pot and moved back into the street, making him miss us when he threw its contents. Shortly after, he came out, mumbling words at us that we couldn't understand as he walked past us toward the police station half a block away. He returned in ten minutes with two carabinieri who asked for our instruments. We could redeem them next day.

My mother's cousin, Commendatore (a title given by the king to someone who has done a great deed for his town) Vassallo, taking his usual evening walk and noticing the commotion, approached us and asked me what had happened. I told him all in detail. He offered to get our instruments back, on the condition that we go to his house and play for an hour. We agreed. Commendatore Vassallo told the carabinieri to return our instruments. He would be responsible for us. We went to Vassallo's. His maid brought us freshly baked cookies and cordials, making it a beautiful evening for all of us—except for the young man who had gone home disappointed.

Another incident during our summer vacation at Shili Sotto occurred when we hired a mason to work on the exterior wall and roof of our house. His name was Vincenzo, and he played guitar and sang. One evening he asked me if I would play my violin as he played the guitar and serenaded a girl who lived nearby.

After supper at dusk we started walking toward the girl's house. As we neared the property, instead of using the path to the house, he decided to cross through vineyards. When we were about seventy-five feet from the house—already dark—Vincenzo said we should start playing, beginning with the song "Oh Mari," as the girl's name was Maria. In two minutes the door opened and out came two barking dogs. We

MY LAST SMALL GAME HUNT IN SICILY

I was due to return to New York early in January 1935 because Italy appeared to be planning to go to war. Uncle Francesco offered to take me and a friend of his on a special hunt before I left. I loved to hunt, especially with him; he taught me all I knew.

The property Francesco took us to was four hours away by donkey. We left at 5:00 P.M. on Friday on three donkeys, each donkey with a dog walking alongside, tied to the right side of the saddle. Donkeys and dogs were trained to this way. At 7:00 we arrived at a farm owned by my parents, where we stayed the night.

The next morning, it was pouring rain. We had a delicious breakfast of sausage and eggs with large mugs of strong coffee. Finally, we set out, wearing hooded ponchos and rubber boots. The donkeys and dogs had a hard time during our two hours in the rain.

On our arrival, the rain diminished. We were greeted

turned and ran. I got tangled in a grapevine, and my violin and bow went flying. Suddenly we heard the father of the girl call the dogs. Then he called to us to come into the house, where we played with Vincenzo singing, and were treated to cordials and cookies. Luckily, Maria's father liked Vincenzo, or it would have been a bad experience. That's the chance you take with serenades.

During the month of September 1933, Connie was coming to term. My mother and Connie were brought home from Shili Sotto, so that when the time came, Connie would have all the help she needed on a moment's notice. I remained, because it was grape-picking time. My job was to bring the grapes by donkey, with one large bamboo basket on each side, to the cement pits where the crushing of the grapes was done. The men would stomp on them, making the juice run into a lower cement pit and leaving the stems, which were put on a press-like contraption. When the grapes were completely squeezed, we put the wine in large sacks made of animal hide, to be emptied into barrels at the final destination to ferment for a few weeks. After the fermentation, it was put into special barrels for aging. During fermentation, the barrels were placed upright with no cork. For aging, the barrels were on their sides with the cork placed lightly in if the wine still fizzled, and closed tightly when the fermentation stopped.

On the morning of September 28, a friend coming out from the town told me that Connie had started labor. Immediately, I set out for town on foot. It took one hour with shortcuts, as opposed to two hours by donkey. Connie went into labor about 8:00 P.M., and shortly after midnight, on September 29, Vincenza came into this world. We gave Vincenza the middle name Cristina, in memory of my grandmother, who had died in August.

Vincenza was a big, healthy baby, weighing about nine pounds. She was the princess of the house, whom everyone catered to. My Grandfather Pasquale arrived daily, climbing the twenty-five steps to our apartment to hold her in his arms, calling her *"Mia batissa"* (my special one).

At the end of the grape season, we began looking around for a farm to buy. There was a fine farm in the county of LaDona outside Caltagirone, twenty-five miles from Licodia Eubea. The property was owned by a minor whose father, on his death, had willed it to him. The boy's guardian decided that it would be wise to sell

warmly by my uncle's friend Massaro Roberto, the owner of the property. (*Massaro* is a Sicilian term for gentleman farmer.) He embraced my uncle. They kissed each other on both cheeks.

The weather was misty. This was ideal for hunting, because the dogs could follow scent much better than they could in dry conditions. While hunting along an orange grove, I spotted a little tree with eight large ripe oranges. Massaro Roberto had told me to pick anything I liked, so I picked one. It was so delicious that I continued picking oranges until the tree was bare of fruit. These are the things you do when you are twenty-three years old.

The hunting was excellent. We bagged sixteen rabbits and ten grouse.

The next day, we were up at dawn. We changed our undergarments, shirt, and socks, and then pulled up a cold pail of water from the well in front of the barn to wash our faces and hands. Breakfast was freshly made cheese, sausage, olives, bread, and wine. We started our second day of hunting on different ground; Massaro Roberto had more than one thousand acres of land. While hunting, we came upon large mushrooms that had sprung up overnight because of the rain, each mushroom weighing nearly half a pound. We now began hunting mushrooms instead of rabbits and grouse. By noon, we had picked nearly fifty pounds of mushrooms, returning to the barn for bushel baskets to put them in. At times, the dogs who continued to hunt would chase a rabbit toward us, making it necessary to shoot, to fulfill the end of the chase for the dogs.

By early afternoon we had four rabbits. We left for home with the two bushels of game and two bushels of mushrooms on our donkeys.

On the four-hour trip home, combined with the slow gait of the donkeys and lots of wine, we dozed often. We arrived home at 7:30, our relatives eagerly waiting for rabbits and grouse. They were pleasantly surprised to see the mushrooms, which were a delicacy. It was a happy time for all.

the property and put the proceeds in trust for the boy's education. After a price was agreed on, it was to be reviewed by the courts of the tribunal to see that the price was sufficient to protect the minor.

The next day, my father, Uncle Francesco, and I went to see this farm. We liked it a great deal. It was the best property of its size in all the territory of Licodia Eubea. The following day, we went to see the guardian, Dr. Russo. He said that the property was part of his soul and he loved it very much. He would sell it only to people who would be worthy of owning the property, but he had great respect for my father. He informed us that a fair price for the farm was 30,000 lires a tumolo. The property was 98 tumoli (worth about $10,000 at the time). We agreed.

What made this property wonderful was that every inch was excellent land. Normally there would be a lot of useless land. About 70 percent was used for wheat, on 10 percent grew two thousand vines of choice eating grapes, and the remaining 20 percent nurtured olive, orange, tangerine, lemon, and walnut trees. There was a house and an enclosure in back for five hundred sheep. We also planned to raise chickens.

The ground floor of the house had four large rooms that were used for stables, supplies, seeds, and other needs. In the center, there was a stairway to a four-room apartment above with a terrace that overlooked the whole property at its highest point. At the far end of the property, a brook ran parallel to our land. On the other side of the brook, there was a large estate with olive trees, owned by a nobleman from Caltagirone. The brook flowed year-round with runoff from the mountains. The lower lands near the brook provided the best quail hunting I ever had.

We planted wheat in the spring and harvested it in August. The harvesting was done by hand with a scythe, then the wheat was put on cleared ground in a circle about twenty-five feet in diameter. A horse or mule was harnessed within the circle and the farmer stood in the center, urging the animal to trot around and around, stamping the wheat so that the grain fell out of its cover. Then the farmer picked up all the wheat, separated it from the foliage, and put it in a large tin colander about two feet in diameter. He shook the colander over a large cloth and the wheat fell through the holes, leaving the wheat chaff in the colander, clean and ready to be put in sacks. This process had to be performed several times until all the grain had been separated.

After the harvest, we planted vegetables, damming the brook to irrigate the fields. Shepherds rented the enclosure in back of the house for their sheep. After the harvest, they grazed some on our land. Our payment for this service was cheese. When fresh, it was soft and delicious, eaten alone or with bread. Aged, it became hard and perfect for grating. We sold what we couldn't use.

5

IN the fall of 1934, we were very concerned about rumors of a war. Even though I had papers protecting me from being called for military service until March 1935, they would not protect me in the event of a war. Everyone was sure we would fight the Germans. By December, the fear of war had hit a high pitch. We decided to return to New York until it blew over.

We telephoned Vincent Palmieri and asked him to book passage for us to New York. We also called friends in Brooklyn, asking them to rent a six-room apartment for us, furnished only with necessities. We would buy the furniture ourselves when we returned. They had an apartment ready for us early in January 1935. We moved in with my parents and one-year-old Vincenza.

My ex-boss, Rocco Quarato, wanted me back, intending to fire my friend Virgil Interligi, to whom I had given my job. I turned down the offer. I couldn't be responsible for Virgil losing his job. But I said I would work in the vacant chair on a commission basis. I was confident that I could build a clientele within a few months.

Rocco refused, and a few days later he fired Virgil, hoping that now I would change my mind. But that was out of the question. Instead I went around the corner to another barbershop. The owner, Paul, offered me a job, provided that I got Rocco's permission. But Rocco said, "Nothing doing. Either you work here or no place nearby. If he hires you, we will be enemies." Under the circumstances, Paul had to refuse. He and Rocco had always been friends.

So the following Monday morning, I went to see Mr. Speciale. In the last two years, times had changed. The agency was filled with barbers waiting for jobs, playing checkers and cards to pass the time. There were at most four calls a day for a barber.

Mr. Speciale called me into his tiny office. All he could offer me was a job on Thirty-third Street and Sixth Avenue. It paid $10 a week with commission. Eager for work, I took the job. The owner was a young man of Italian descent. He was planning to sell the shop to Izzy, a Jewish barber who worked there.

I wasn't too happy the first week, but Izzy urged me to stick it out until he took over the shop in three weeks. He promised that things would be better for me. When he finally took over the shop two months later, Izzy insisted that I work in the first chair. He remained in the second, installing a new barber in the third chair that I had once occupied. He was aware that customers believed that the barber in the first chair was the boss, and so they did not tip me. When I quit and began packing my barber tools, Izzy offered me the second chair. But I didn't like his principles, nor did I trust him. So I left.

Monday morning, I was back in Mr. Speciale's office. He knew what had happened because Izzy had called him for a barber. Mr. Speciale said that I had done the right thing. He had one job for me. It paid $18 a week, possibly with a $5 to $10 commission, and approximately $12 to $15 in tips. But the shop was one of the best in the city.

I went promptly to the Lorraine Barber Shop at 545 Fifth Avenue, on the corner of Forty-fifth Street. The shop was in the lobby. This was the job I had dreamed about. I was stopped by an elderly gentleman as I walked in. He was the "brush boy" at the hat rack near the entrance. He asked me what I wanted. Obviously, I didn't look like a customer, but I looked too young to be a barber. I showed him the paper from the Speciale agency. He pointed out a leather sofa and told me to sit down. As soon as the boss, Mr. Tarantino, was free, he would talk to me.

The shop had eight barbers, six facing the entrance and one on each side of the shop. The manager was on the left and the owner on the right. The shop was beautifully furnished and air-conditioned, a rarity in those days. As I waited, I began to get cold feet. I

THE ADDICTED NOSE WITH THE EXPENSIVE SNEEZE

Henrik Van Loon was a writer and historian who wrote from the late 1920s until his death in 1944. He was a big man, about six foot six and 300 pounds. He was addicted to a tickling sensation on his nose from my vibrator during a facial massage, which made him sneeze. He said sneezing helped him think better. He came in for a massage three or four times a week. His normal tip for a massage was 50¢, and he added 10¢ for each sneeze, sometimes sneezing as many as ten times.

When he lay down in the barber chair, he was so big that his feet hung in the sink. When he sneezed, it thundered the shop. The barbers waited for the sneezes, calling out, "one," "two," "three," with each sneeze. Even other clients would join in. When he was sneezed out, he lifted his hand to notify you to stop.

One day, seven of the eight

barbers were busy, with the eighth barber not in, and that day Mr. Van Loon said he needed a massage. I put him in the empty chair, telling my barbers to work on him if they had a late appointment, taking up where the last barber left off, until their appointment came in. Five barbers, each giving about five minutes of his time, gave him the massage, which took about an hour, as Van Loon had to wait five to ten minutes between barbers. Of course, Mr. Van Loon was very happy and appreciative, giving 50¢ each to the five barbers and $1 to me for conceiving the idea.

Unfortunately, two days later, Henrik Van Loon died of a heart attack. Five barbers might have been too much for him. The motto of this account is, "Never let more than one barber tend to your tonsorial needs."

was losing my nerve, but I was ashamed to go past the brush boy. After fifteen minutes, Mr. Tarantino finished with his client. He walked up to me, introduced himself, and asked for my slip of paper that Mr. Speciale had given me. Reading it, he said, "Everything is okay except the hours. They are nine to seven, not eight to seven. We have two shifts. Go in that closet and fit yourself a pair of white pants and a jacket. There is your chair, so get to work." I couldn't believe my ears. He didn't ask me a single question. This had never happened before.

Happy and nervous, I put on my uniform and went to chair number six. Putting my tools in order, I was ready to work within ten minutes. Immediately, Mr. Tarantino sent me a customer for a haircut. I was nervous and confessed to the man that he was my first customer. When I finished, the customer said to Mr. Tarantino, "You have a good barber there. Please give me his card." (Incidentally, I took care of this client for forty-seven years, until my retirement. His name was Gus Rundbaken.)

The system in the shop was very different. Mr. Tarantino told me to pay attention to the other barbers to learn the shop technique of facial massages and scalp treatments. Also, I was not to read magazines or newspapers in my spare time. I should be devoted solely to picking up the system. Moreover, if I weren't busy, I was not to walk around the chair or shop unless I wanted to go to the men's room or use the telephone booths in the lobby.

The shop was busy, and I didn't have many opportunities to learn by watching. I was sure of myself giving shaves and haircuts, but I made many mistakes giving massages. Every time I looked up, I would see the manager, Joe Gallo, or Mr. Tarantino staring at me. I expected to be fired at any time.

But on my fourth day on the job, when I had just finished with a client, Mr. Gallo came and told me that Mr. Tarantino was downstairs in the restaurant waiting to speak to me. As I opened the door to the restaurant, I noticed Mr. Tarantino sitting with two coffees and two portions of apple pie. As I sat down, Mr. Tarantino said, "What the fuck is the matter with you? Why are you so nervous?" I let out a big sigh of relief. Then I slowly told him of the good job I had when I got married, what had happened to me since, and how much I wanted this job. But not

FACIAL MASSAGE

First, apply cocoa butter cream to the face with relaxing hand movements for circulation of blood, for two minutes.

Place a hot towel from the sterilizer gently over the face for about thirty seconds. Then apply the vibrator gently over the hot towel, using slight pressure, to four specific areas of the face. With very fluid and gentle motions, and while keeping one hand in contact with the client's face at all times, fold a clean towel to wipe excess cream off the client's face.

Discard the towel and for five minutes continue slowly to massage the face, scalp, and shoulders for relaxation and to circulate blood to the head.

Next, apply Pompain cream and massage it into the face until it rolls off any grease remaining from the cocoa butter.

Apply a fresh hot towel to remove any remaining grease from face, ears, and neck.

Saturate one-third of the end of a linen towel with Dickinson Witch Hazel, placing the wet end over the face below the mouth. Then rub the forehead and temples with Orage Rub (mentholated liquid) and cover it with the remaining part of towel saturated with witch hazel.

Put drops of Murine in each eye, opening and closing eyes with a finger, then place a piece of absorbent cotton over the eyes and re-cover with witch hazel–soaked towel, leaving nose uncovered. Place two steamed hot towels over witch hazel–soaked towel, one over the other. Then saturate a piece of cotton with Orage Rub and put under nose, leaving sufficient room for the client to breathe freely.

Apply the vibrator over the hot towel, using slight pressure on three or four spots for thirty seconds.

Have cold towel from refrigerator ready, folded lengthwise. Remove all towels from the face and toss into the sink. Immediately apply cold towel over forehead and ears for ten seconds, then pat the entire face with it.

Finish off with any aftershave or cologne desired.

having the experience for an excellent shop, I feared I would be let go from one minute to the next. In fact, I thought this was the end. He laughed and said, "I knew you were the barber I wanted after your first two customers by the way you handled your razor, scissors, and comb. You are as good as any barber upstairs. No one is going to fire you." I went back upstairs with great confidence. Within six months, I grossed as much as barbers who had been there for eight or ten years.

At the end of 1936, Barbers Union Local No. 1 representatives came to the shop daily to try to unionize us. They waited for us outside when we went to lunch or went home, as Mr. Tarantino wouldn't allow them to come into the shop to talk to us. One of the barbers who was defiant was beaten up on his way home. I was the most junior employee, so I told the older barbers that whatever they did, I would do. Mr. Tarantino had a meeting with us, saying that he ran the best shop in New York City, had the best conditions, one-week vacations, and air-conditioning for our comfort and for the shop's success. We had also profited handsomely in commissions and tips. If we joined the union, he would sell the shop.

After two difficult months, the shop was unionized. Mr. Tarantino called a meeting and was furious, saying he didn't need a union to tell him how to run his shop. Two months later, Mr. Tarantino sold the shop to Ernest Bivona, the worst shop manager I have ever seen in my barbering career.

Bivona's daily ritual was to come in at 10:00 A.M., wearing striped pants and solid blue jacket with a fresh carnation in his lapel. First he greeted the manager on his left, then he went down the line, from chair to chair, saying good morning to each barber individually with a big smile. Then Bivona went to the cash register and counted the morning's receipts, after which he came to my chair for a shave. He had been told I was a superb shaver, probably because I had mastered the art of honing my razor to perfection.

In those days, a sharp razor made a good shaver. Very few barbers mastered the art of honing a razor. A well-honed razor not only enabled you to do more shaves, but it was also smoother and sweeter, as we called it.

HONING AND STROPPING A RAZOR

The razor first has to be honed on a soapstone. A soapstone hones better and the sharp edge lasts longer if shaving soap is applied for the honing process. Hence, the name. If done without soap, the razor isn't as smooth when sharpened and doesn't last more than two or three shaves. If soap is used and if the barber has mastered the honing process, it can do fifteen shaves and sometimes more, depending on the individual razor's steel quality.

A shaving razor needs the finishing touch of a stropping on a piece of heavy linen, usually three inches by eighteen inches. This gives the razor a better edge. The leather strop of soft cowhide is then used to smooth and finish the rough edge. The stropping process is repeated for every half a face shaved.

A razor that was not honed to perfection didn't feel as smooth and at times even pulled the beard before cutting, making it uncomfortable and painful. A good barber sometimes spent two or three hours honing his set

MR. MONTMARTAN, THE FRENCHMAN WITH A SHADY PAST

I met Mr. Montmartan in the spring of 1939. He had rented a small office in the building where my first barber shop was located, at 535 Fifth Avenue. After introducing himself and complimenting me on a beautiful shop, he proceeded to tell me the services he required. He would come for a shave twice a day at about 10:00 A.M. and 5:00 P.M., a sunlamp treatment every other day, a haircut every Saturday, and a shampoo and manicure on Wednesday and Saturday. After each shampoo, he wanted his hair saturated with Chanel No. 5 (he would bring a large bottle, for his personal use only), a finger wave (to make his hair look thicker), and a hair net put over it for drying. When dry, he wanted it combed out. I couldn't believe my ears. He left telling me that his secretary would call me for an appointment. Next morning, his male secretary called for a 10:00 A.M. ap-

of razors with a good soapstone, which was difficult to get.

Today, barbers have no razor problems because they can buy excellent presharpened blades. They insert them in a razor handle, replacing them when they start faltering. Today's barber, having this convenience, doesn't know how to use a razor for shaving, except a safety razor.

After his shave, Mr. Bivona wanted a good scalp rub with Eau De Quinine hair tonic and his hair parted and combed to perfection. Then he would get out of the chair, looking at himself in the mirror, and say, "Very good, Pat. Thank you." He always gave me a 25¢ tip and requested a check for his services. He then walked around the shop full of smiles.

He became edgy about 11:30. Sometime between 11:30 and noon, he would get a phone call and then go out. He would return by 4:00 P.M. and walk straight to the leather sofa that waiting customers used. He would sit in a corner, close his eyes, and fall asleep. He woke up at 6:00, checked the receipts for the day, and closed the shop at 7:00. The shop was getting worse and worse, order to disorder.

One day, Bivona's wife came in about 1:00 P.M. On being told that her husband was out and would be back at about 4:00, she said, "I know where he is!" and left in a rage. The following day, Mr. Bivona came in, as usual, at 10:00 A.M. His face was swollen, with black and blue marks. He didn't say his usual individual good mornings, and he sat in my chair for his usual shave in silence. The next morning, his brother-in-law told us what had happened.

Bivona had a girlfriend who was a manicurist at the Commodore Hotel, where he once had worked. She worked the early shift and went home at noon. She called Mr. Bivona when she was ready to leave, and he picked her up in a cab and took her to her apartment, where he stayed until he returned to the shop at 4:00. Mrs. Bivona became suspicious and had him followed by a friend. She found out all she needed to know, including the girl's address. After leaving our shop the day before, she had gone to the manicurist's apartment. When the girl opened the door slightly to see who it was, Mrs. Bivona, who was a strong woman, pushed her aside, exposing Ernest in the kitchen with an apron on and a skillet in his hands.

pointment. After that, he came as regularly as he had said.

As time went on, I found out more and more about this unusual individual. He was extremely conceited, looking down on everyone. He hated Jews. Money was his God, and he felt he could buy anyone with it. His wife and two daughters often traveled to South America and Australia, and he always had one or two French models following him wherever he went. I came to the point of hating him. But I needed his $25 a week.

In the building, we had a bootblack who went from office to office to shine shoes. His name was Jimmy. He'd been a victim of poison gas in World War I as a U.S. soldier, so he couldn't hold down a job. He was so well liked in the building that tenants took up a collection for him to visit his brother in Naples, whom he always spoke of. When Mr. Montmartan first moved into the building, Jimmy opened his door and said, "Shine?" Mr. Montmartan yelled, "Get out of here! Never come here again. You dirty my office!"

One rainy day, Mr. Montmartan came into the building and into the elevator full of people. Who should walk into the elevator but Jimmy with his shoeshine box. He had shined shoes in the stores on the ground floor. As the elevator started up, Mr. Montmartan looked down at Jimmy (Montmartan was six feet tall and Jimmy only five foot one) and said, "Come to my office and clean my shoes."

Jimmy looked up at him and said, "I will not. I don't want to dirty my brushes on your dirty shoes." Mr. Montmartan, embarrassed and furious, said nothing.

Later, a client of the shop who knew Montmartan spoke to his wife about him. She was working for a magazine that was doing an article on people exploiting Jews running from Hitler by buying their valuables cheaply. One of these buyers turned out to be Montmartan, a Jew himself who had changed his name from Solomon. He was known to have bought paintings from desperate Jews for a fraction of their worth, then taken them

She grabbed the skillet and started hitting him on the face and head, yelling, "At home you never go near the stove, but here you become a cook." When she was through with him, she threw the skillet at the girl, just missing her, and left, shouting, "You can keep him!"

About a month later, we were notified that the shop had been sold to Barney Penn. He owned a barbershop and beauty parlor at 551 Fifth Avenue, in the French Building, as well as two others in the vicinity. Barney Penn had more vices than Ernest Bivona ever had: women, betting on horses, and gambling of every sort. He took over the shop's mortgage of $2,000 and paid $1,000 cash for the shop. Only months before, it had cost Ernest Bivona $8,000.

On November 25, 1937, Thanksgiving Day, Connie had our second daughter, Katherine. She was named after Connie's mother. Connie hated to miss Thanksgiving and all the holiday food she and my mother had prepared. So we all brought samples of everything to the hospital.

Jack Sciarabba, a barber who had worked in the shop for six months, had opened his own shop at 535 Fifth

Avenue, a block away. He had been forced to close the shop when a very substantial tenant moved out of the building and he lost about 75 percent of his clients. Now that space was being taken over by Russian War Relief, the OPA, and the Selective Service headquarters for New York City. They attracted nowhere near the quality of clientele of the previous tenant, but Jack asked me if I would like to reopen his shop as partners. I wasn't happy working for Penn, so I agreed. Albert, another of Penn's barbers, who had an excellent following, wanted to come work for us. With the strong following we all had, we felt we couldn't go wrong.

through Spain and Portugal to the United States, where he sold them for their true value.

When I went to Susca's other shop, 90 percent of my clients came with me. I had too many clients to take care of, so Mr. Susca decided it was time to rid myself of Mr. Montmartan. The next morning when his secretary called for his usual appointment, I said, "Tell Mr. Montmartan to find himself another barber. Pat has no more time for him." Not believing his secretary, Montmartan himself called right back. I told him the same thing and hung up.

I never saw him again, which made me very happy.

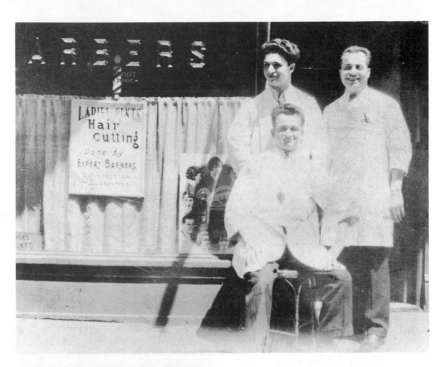

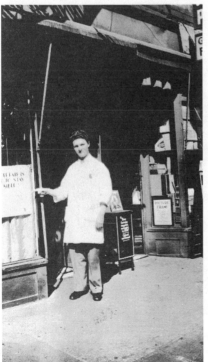

Above: Rocco's Barber Shop in 1930. From left to right: me, Nicola Puglisi, and Rocco Quarato.

Left: Working at Rocco's Barber Shop in 1929. I was eighteen years old.

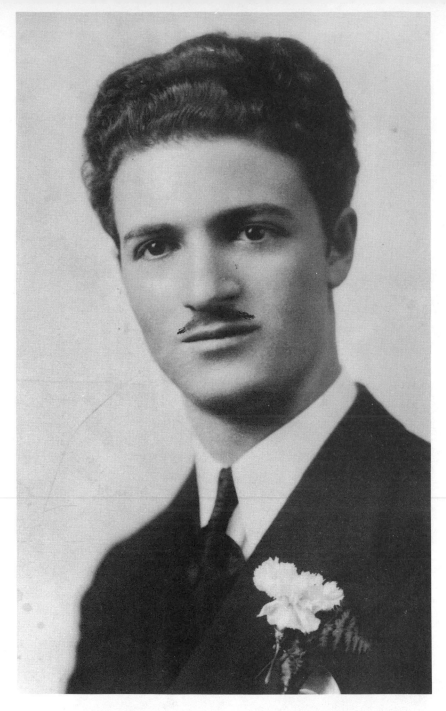

Here I am upon my engagement to Connie in September 1931.

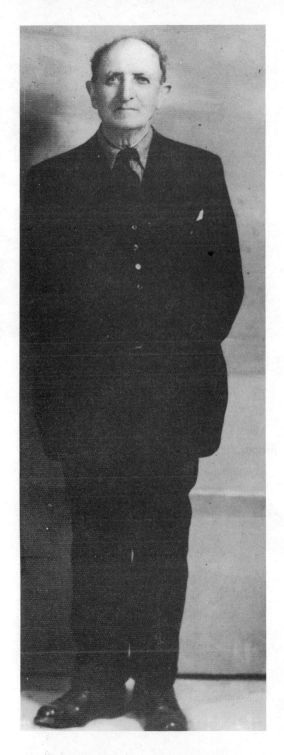

My maternal uncle,
Francesco Vassallo.

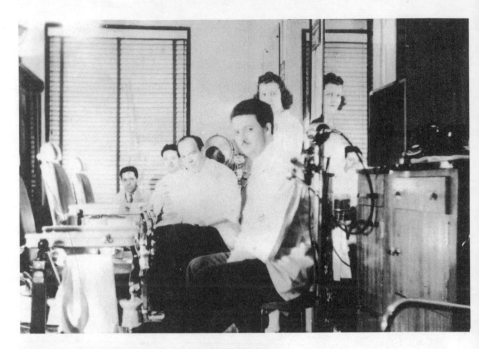

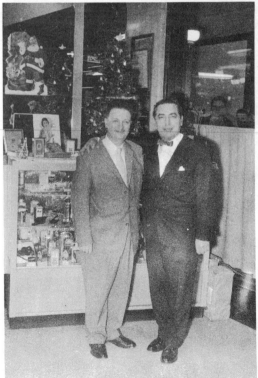

Above: The staff of my first establishment, the Rupert Building Barber Shop.

Left: Angelo Copertino on my left in 1960 at the Arcade Barber Shop.

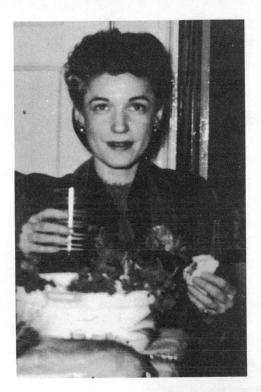

Left: Hilda Withrow, the manicurist at the Arcade Barber Shop.

Below: Hilda Withrow doing a manicure at the Arcade Barber Shop. I'm giving a haircut.

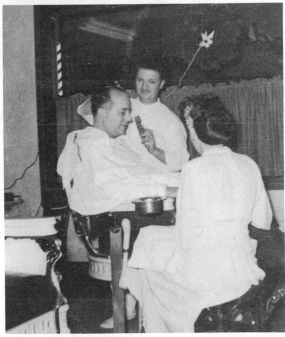

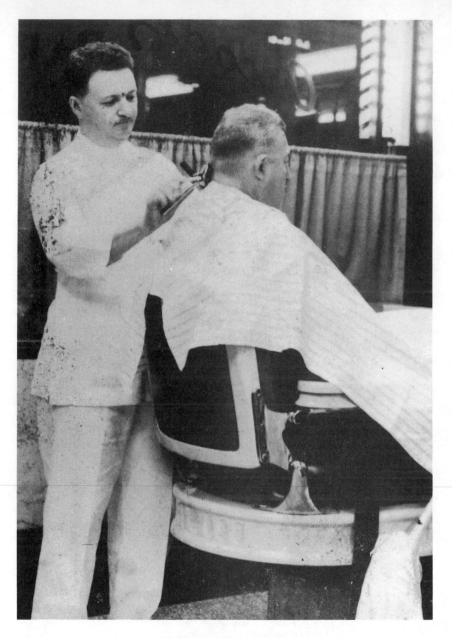

Above and opposite, top: Working at the Arcade Barber Shop.

Opposite, bottom: A view of the Arcade Barber Shop as it looked in 1968. I'm standing in the center of the shop with my partner Angelo Copertino at my left.

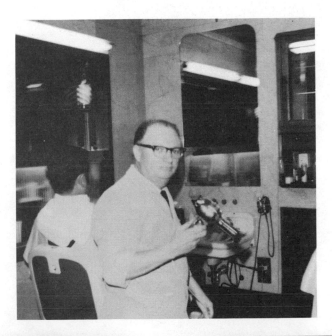

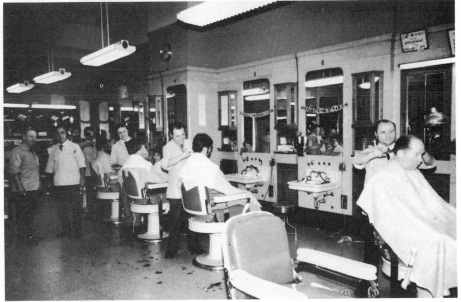

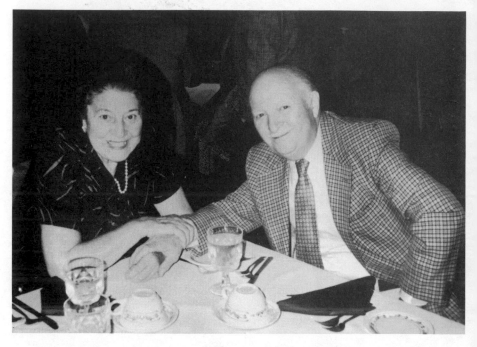

My wife, Connie, with me in 1987 on my seventy-sixth birthday.

6

IN May 1938, we opened our fifth-floor shop. The shop was beautiful, with new, modern fixtures. During the first two weeks, all of Jack's and my clients arrived. But only about 35 percent of Albert's came. Albert became discouraged. Barney Penn, noticing that Albert's customers were still coming to his shop, often waited outside the building at night to meet Albert. He would take him for a drink, telling him which of his customers had come into the shop. Albert, with a wife and four children, gradually became convinced to go back. We begged him to give it another week, but couldn't change his mind. Naturally, in the third week, Albert's customers started calling for appointments. We had to tell them that Albert had gone back to the Lorraine Barber Shop.

Jack and I remained alone, working very hard, and advertising to increase business. We added another barber in two months. I took home $30 less per week, even though we paid only $40 rent per month. Jack was happy: He was fifty-five years old, and his children

A RABBIT DILEMMA

At the Lorraine Barber Shop, we had a manicurist named Adeline Dawn. She was from Birmingham, Alabama, and had a beautiful southern accent. She was well endowed, blond, pretty, intelligent, and had a beautiful personality.

Adeline's favorite topic with clients was when she would retire. She wanted to run a rabbit farm. She had all the figures about how fast rabbits multiply. The clients who knew this always brought up the subject for a few laughs, asking Adeline when the rabbit farm was going to be started.

Jack Gimbel told her one day he was going to get her started with imported rabbits that weighed almost ten pounds each. This went on for a period, then one morning a truck driver from a Railway Express truck came in the shop asking for Miss Adeline Dawn, saying that he had a crate full of rabbits to deliver to her, sent by a Mr. Jack Gimbel.

Adeline, thinking fast, told

were already working. But I was only twenty-seven. I realized the mistakes I had made: going into business with someone twice my age, and opening a shop on the fifth floor. In our eagerness to go into business, we had invested $2,000, and I was reluctant to give it up.

In 1940, Jack decided to sell his share to a barber working for us, Frank Chiodo. The war was getting closer and closer. In May of 1941, our lease expired. A few months later, Frank was called up by the army. Then I got a fifteen-day notice to vacate the shop because the Russian War Relief Committee needed the entire fifth floor. I kissed the notice forcing me to vacate. Barney Penn, knowing the situation, came to me and offered me the opportunity to manage his shop at 521 Fifth Avenue. I told him that since I could bring all the clientele from my shop, I wanted to be compensated for it. Also, I wanted to have the right to hire and fire, as he did all the hiring and firing in his other shops. He said he couldn't give me terms different from the other managers.

Then I had an idea. I went to a barbershop half a block away at 19 West Forty-fourth Street, an eight-chair shop with beautiful fixtures made of

Italian marble. It was owned by Joseph Susca, who was in his sixties. After introducing myself and filling him in on my situation, I asked him if he would rent me the last chair. There were five barbers and three empty chairs. I told him I didn't need clients from his shop because I had many of my own, and he could have the gross from my manicure business, which had about thirty clients weekly. As it happened, he had too much business for his one manicurist, but not enough for two. He liked my proposition. I demanded a contract that specified that he give me three months' notice to fire me, but that I could leave at any time. He agreed. Also, I would charge my own prices (they were higher than his on certain items) and make my own hours. The shop was open from eight to seven. I came in at nine and went home at six.

I now was in business for myself with no responsibilities for rent, electricity, and the like. I was both happy and proud of the deal I had struck, and Mr. Susca was equally elated. His manicure problems were over; the shop was busier, giving it a shot in the arm that made a noticeable difference. He netted about 15 percent of my gross plus his profit on the manicurist. I tripled my take-home pay,

the truck driver that the rabbits were supposed to be delivered to her home, giving the address of a gentleman friend, Harold Peet. She told the driver that she would get a cab and be home when he got there. When the truck arrived, Adeline had all the rabbits put in the bathroom. She then came back to the shop. When her friend came home from his office, he opened the bathroom door and was almost run out of the apartment by rabbits wanting to get out. He quickly came to his senses, pushing them back in and closing the door, completely forgetting his need of the bathroom.

Coming to the conclusion that Adeline was the culprit— only she had a key to his apartment—he called her at the shop, giving her hell for the rabbits. Adeline told him that she would be there shortly to explain and help solve the mess that she had created. On her arrival, Harold was still furious, saying he had to use the next-door neighbor's bathroom. After Adeline calmed him down some, they debated what to do. Looking at each other, they both began to laugh, coming to the conclusion that the bathroom, with its slippery floor, wasn't the best place to start a rabbit farm. They wouldn't mate and multiply there. Harold decided to call the super of the building to see if he could help solve their problem. The super, a German immigrant who loved rabbit meat, said he would be happy to take them all. He solved the rabbit dilemma.

thanking God for the fifteen-day notice that I received to vacate the fifth-floor barber shop.

I met Angelo Copertino at Mr. Susca's shop. Angelo worked on the fifth chair, the one closest to me. He was the busiest and the best barber in the shop. We became good friends as we were almost the same age. A year later, Angelo was notified by his draft board that unless he stopped barbering and went into defense work, he would be drafted. He had two children and a wife, Margaret, so of course he immediately quit and found himself a job in a defense factory. Angelo was older than me, but he had been notified first because his wife worked; she could support the family, if necessary. Frank Chiodo, older than both of us, was inducted because both he and his wife worked, with no children to support.

At around this time, Connie gave birth to our third daughter. We named her Frances, after my father. Frances was tiny, and her sisters adored her. They thought they had been given a little doll. My standard answer to anyone who asked, "What was it?" was "As usual." Connie and I gave up on having a boy.

Early in 1945, I heard about a barbershop for sale across the street in the lobby of 28 West Forty-fourth Street that went through to 25 West Forty-third Street. It had eight chairs with five manned. On my next visit to Angelo, I told him about it. He was very interested. He kept telling me that when the war ended, we could buy the shop together. I had exactly the same idea. We both looked forward to it.

After a few months, when the war ended, we went to see the owner, Albert Argentieri. He had owned his barbershop for twenty-five years. It was run-down, dilapidated and dingy, with three very old barbers who had little to offer but good workmanship. This is not enough for a successful barbershop; it accounts for only about 35 percent. The other 65 percent is personality and know-how. The owner was just a nice guy. We bargained with Mr. Argentieri for one week. Finally, we agreed to pay $3,000 now and $3,000 within two years.

We took possession of the Arcade Barber Shop, so named because it was in the main arcade of the building, in June of 1945. Angelo quit his defense job where he had worked for two years. I just moved across the street. Mr. Susca was very angry with us, even though it was my own clientele that I took, no clients from his shop. Mr. Susca was even angrier with Angelo, primarily because they were family friends who came from Conversano in the province of Bari. But Angelo had been away from the shop for two years, and most of his clients were already used to other barbers.

Angelo contacted only the clients who weren't going to Susca's anymore. Some came, others didn't. We wanted to go into business for ourselves, not put Susca out of business. Of course, all my old clients came to the new location. Angelo took over all of Mr. Argentieri's clients, plus new customers who were not going to Mr. Susca's shop. The youngest barber there was seventy years old; the oldest barber was eighty-four and the best of the lot. They protested our new regulations, especially raising prices. We put new mirrors in and twice as many lights. We stopped clients from making appointments for only a free mustache or beard trim between haircuts. We also stopped clients from making appointments with no charge to have their nails cleaned between manicures, even though the barber or manicurist was compensated with a tip.

We immediately realized that the seventy-year-old was not a good barber, especially with haircuts. We fired him after the first week. We later found out that prior to working there, he had worked in the Tombs (the city jail). It was the price you paid for hiring a barber during the war when there were few barbers to be had. Two others who had been there more than ten years thought that our new regulations would cost them their clients. So they found jobs in the Barney Penn shops, taking clients with them. The eighty-four-year-old, John La Motte, was stone deaf and had been there more than twenty years. He worked with us for another year until health problems forced him to retire.

It was difficult after the war to find good beginners and teach them the fine points of the trade. The first barber we hired was Angelo's brother-in-law, Jimmy L'Abbato. He had begun barbering before the war and cut hair in the army. He had an excellent personality and was very ambitious. In short order, with our help and his efforts, he became a first-class barber. While training Jimmy, we hired another young man with the same qualifications, who had been in the navy. He was also an excellent choice. He had a super personality.

We continued hiring young men, with excellent results. Our problems with help involved getting good manicurists. We put up with a few until we found good, experienced operators. We progressed steadily, doing what had to be done. Our barbers and manicurists always gave us respect as their superiors and appreciated what we had done for them. I put in practice everything I had learned from Dan Tarantino during the short time I had worked for him. He was the best boss I've ever seen in fifty-five years of barbering.

About this time, we employed a manicurist whose name was Hilda Withrow. After hiring her, we learned about her interesting background. It honored me to cross her path. She had been an orphan from the age of ten, living in Middletown, Ohio. She and a brother who was partly paralyzed were taken in by relatives. Their intention was to work her as a slave, having her do all kinds of chores around the house, manual and otherwise. She realized that she had to do her best to please them so that she and her younger brother would survive. As she became older, she took correspondence courses in writing, sewing, millinery, detective work, and others. But her ambition was to be a writer.

When she was eighteen years old, she decided to go to Cincinnati. Her brother was able to do the chores, which would allow him to stay on with the relatives. Arriving in Cincinnati, she found a job with the Trinity Paper Bag Company. While there, she took evening classes in beauty culture. When she graduated from beautician's school, she decided to come to New York to work as a beautician and eventually to write. After finding herself an apartment, she got a job as a mani-

HOW WE PROMOTED OUR SERVICE BUSINESS

On a slow day (we could predict a slow day if it was raining or snowing or if a low number of appointments were taken by noon), we would alert the barbers to tell steady clients of theirs who they thought could afford a massage, shampoo, or manicure, but who had never asked for one, that we were offering a free introductory massage, shampoo, or manicure. There were usually five or six clients out of ten who, after receiving the free service once, requested it from then on. The ones who didn't request the extra service every time did ask for it at least now and then.

curist in a barbershop. (She found men easier to work with than women.) Between clients, in her spare time, she could write at her table. Her first job was in a shop on West Thirty-seventh Street in the garment center. After working there for two years, she decided to find a job in a better environment. The clientele often used vulgar language and even made propositions.

Hilda began looking at want ads in the New York *Journal American*. She saw our ad for a manicurist, but she was too timid to come into the shop. About a month later, we ran the ad again, and again she came to the shop but lost her nerve to enter. Luck would have it that about a month later we advertised yet again. This time she came in. I could see that she was uneasy, puffing nervously on her cigarette. As was customary when someone looked to be a good prospect, we took him or her next door for a cup of coffee. In the coffee shop, she immediately told me that this was her third try in three months applying for a job at our shop. But now she was happy that she had come in. And with her experience, we were happy to have her.

She worked out wonderfully. She was intelligent, reliable, an excellent worker, and very much a lady. Seeing that she was always writing when she wasn't busy, we asked her about it. She said, "Someday, I will be a writer." Up until now, she had written only short stories, which she had sent to magazines. All of them were rejected, but she was determined to keep writing until they were accepted.

As time went on, we found out that every evening she had supper at a Horn and Hardart. These restaurants were patronized by people who didn't have much to spend. But they had excellent food, especially coffee and pies. After Hilda put her food on her tray, she always looked around for someone who seemed down on his or her luck, then sat down and started a conversation. She believed she had good judgment, because of her correspondence course in private detective work. If, during the conversation, she felt that someone, male or female, was having hard luck and seemed trustworthy, she often took the person home and fed and clothed him or her. In the meantime, she got the stories of their downfall. She never had a problem with any of the down-and-outers. At times, Hilda would show us a letter she received from someone she had helped. Some sent her a check in appreciation. She loved the work in our shop. It had given her confidence, as many of our clients were officers of large corporations, writers, entertainers, actors, lawyers, and accountants. WINS and *The New Yorker* magazine were in the building.

Early in 1951, Hilda came in one morning very excited. She had won second prize of $500 in a Dr. Christian radio script contest. She asked us if we would be present at the theater where she would receive the prize. Angelo, who wanted to do something special for Hilda, had an idea. We called Joe Rutolo, for whom we had found a job as chauffeur to our client Ward Melville, chairman of the

MANICURING

Manicurists in our shop were told to heed clients' requests, to be pleasant, and to finish manicures with a hand massage using cream. Last but not least, if a new client undertipped (less than a minimum tip that we stipulated), the manicurist should come to us, and we would make up the difference to the manicurist. If that customer came back and continued to undertip, the third time he did so, either Angelo or I would walk out of the shop with him, telling him the problem. Nine out of ten clients thanked us and usually started tipping more. One in ten would get angry and never come into the shop again. If we didn't do this, the client possibly wouldn't get the same attention or quality of work from the manicurist. If we were going to lose a client, we preferred to lose him because he thought we were too expensive, not because he thought our manicurists were not up to standard.

board of Melville Shoes, and told him about Hilda's good fortune. We asked if he were free that evening. He said he was taking Mr. and Mrs. Melville to the opera at 8:00 and would be free after that until 11:00. We told Joe what we had in mind, and he thought it was a fine idea.

When Hilda was presented with her prize check on the stage of the theater, Angelo and I sent two baskets of flowers up to her. We walked toward the exit with Hilda between us, holding the two baskets of flowers in front of her. Out on the street, there was Joe in uniform opening the door of the limousine. Hilda was deeply moved. "You have made me feel like a princess," she said.

Since *The New Yorker* was in the same building as our barbershop, Angelo decided to call one of his clients there to tell him what had happened to Hilda. About a half hour later, Brendan Gill called, saying that he had been told about Hilda and asking if he could come to interview her. We had a one-hour interview by Mr. Gill, whose story appeared in the June 30, 1951, issue. Here it is.

MR. KNOW-HOW

The barbershop in the lobby of our building is owned by a couple of capable fellows named Angelo Copertino and Pat Spagnuolo. Angelo called us up the other day and, in a voice choked with excitement, announced that a script written by Miss Hilda Withrow, one of the three manicurists in the shop, had won a five-hundred-dollar second prize in the Dr. Christian radio contest. "Nice girl, nice manicurist, nice prize," Angelo said, and invited us to have a talk with her. To the best of our knowledge, this is the first time the lightning of radio fortune has ever struck the premises, and we went straight downstairs to interview Miss Withrow. Slender, pleasant-faced, and in her mid-thirties, Miss Withrow gave our cuticles a disapproving glance and said at once that she was sure she had never done *us*. We confessed that though we had our hair cut in the shop regularly, we didn't get manicures. "Some men don't. Lawyers are the neat ones," she said, and then, as if to show that she forgave us, stated that except for our cuticles it would be easy to mistake us for a lawyer. Thus flattered and fortified, we asked Miss Withrow whether she had been writing radio scripts for long. "I've been writing them for years, and never had a single one accepted," she said. " 'Mr. Know-How,' which won the prize, was the tenth script I'd submitted in the Dr. Christian Contests. I also write essays and short stories. I especially like writing short-shorts—not the gimmick ones, the mood ones—But I haven't sold any."

Miss Withrow told us that she is a native of Middletown, Ohio. . . . She got a job in a paper-bag factory, where she spent six unfruitful years. She took a night-school course in "beauty," and in 1940 moved to Cincinnati, where she found work as a hairdresser in a beauty salon. She spent her Cincinnati nights at a dramatic school, with the intention of going on the stage. Rehearsals proved boring, however, and it struck her that playwrights are more to be envied than actors. "The man who writes a play only has to do it once," she said to herself, "but the actor has to do it over and over." This epiphany led her to sit down and dash off a comedy entitled "All in a Day." She mailed it to the New York office of Samuel French, who returned it so fast that it might almost have been intercepted in Pittsburgh. "Mr. French was absolutely right," Miss Withrow said. "I was new to playwriting, and I didn't realize you had to have a plot."

In 1944, Miss Withrow came East, in order to be close to the literary market. For the past five years she has been working as a manicurist in our building during the day and writing every night. She gave up hairdressing because she finds men easier to please than women, and more interesting to talk to. She is not married. When we indicated our surprise, she said the reason that she hadn't married was that she had yet to find a man willing to share all her varied interests, which, besides writing, included music (she is currently taking mandolin lessons at the New York School of Music), intensive reading in philosophy (her favorite authors are Emerson, William James, and Kahlil Gibran), and millinery (she makes her own hats).

Miss Withrow took a correspondence course in radio-script writing, and credits that course with having taught her how to build a story in dialogue and with having trained her in the proper use of radio vernacular, such as "bridge," "sustain to flashback," and "segue to sound." She informed us that the Dr. Christian radio show is broadcast every Wednesday evening over C.B.S. and is the only show on the air that is written by the listening audience. "Most of the scripts are by writers like me, outside the profession," she said. "Every year, a contest is held, and you're supposed to slant your script to fit the homely, small-town philosophy of Dr. Christian, who is Jean Hersholt in real life. Dr. Christian is an old-fashioned family physician and believes that *every*body has something of value to give in this world. The first prize in the contest is two thousand dollars. There are three second prizes of five hundred dollars. Other scripts are bought for a minimum of two hundred fifty dollars. The owner of the first prize this year was a Mr. Fred McWhorter, an insurance man in Kansas City, Missouri. His script, which has already been broadcast, was entitled, "The Home-coming," and Miss Withrow described it as emphasizing patriotism, religion, and tolerance.

Miss Withrow's script, "Mr. Know-How," which will be broadcast later this year, tells of an old man, retired because of a cardiac condition, whose habit of giving unasked-for advice makes him a nuisance to everyone; Dr. Christian straightens him out so deftly that at the end he is the highly paid writer of a newspaper column of advice to perplexed persons. When Miss Withrow went to the broadcasting studio to receive her prize, she found that the two bosses had sent baskets of flowers on ahead of her. Afterward, Angelo and Pat, dressed to the nines, called for her in a chauffeur-driven Cadillac. "They looked beautiful—just like diplomats," she said. "I was so proud. Everybody wondered who I was. I took my flowers home and put them in the icebox, and they kept just fine."

Knowing how carefully she used her money, I talked Hilda into investing the $500 in Mobil Oil stock, where she couldn't touch it. I believed it would increase in value and also pay good dividends. After a few years, she sold the stock, tripling her investment.

Later that year, we had a citywide barber strike. A month earlier, I was shaving Thomas McLoud, president of Stern's department store, whom I shaved daily. Predicting a long strike, I asked him a favor. I told him that I would appreciate it if he would find a job for Hilda in his store, even wrapping packages, just so she had some money to carry her through a couple of months. By this time, all of our customers knew about Hilda's beautiful story. We had blown up *The New Yorker* piece and put it in our window. We were very proud of it. Mr. McLoud looked at me without saying a

BY THE BLUEPRINT
OF A BEARD

One day a new client came in and said that he would like a shave. I lowered the chair to a shaving position and prepared him, putting on a clean towel after washing my hands, then rubbing a little Noxzema shaving cream on his beard (as a base for the lather), a steamed hot towel over, stropping my razor, then taking off the hot towel, putting lather over the beard, and rubbing until the beard was ready to shave.

When I finished the right side, I stopped. I said, "Sir, this has never happened to me in all my years of barbering." Looking worried, he asked me what was wrong. I said, "You have a beard just like Moe Behrman, whom I shaved daily for over twenty years, until he died two years ago. You have the same grain and just as tough a beard as he had. His was the toughest." Smiling, he said, "Yes, I know. I'm his brother Sam. My other brother, Harry, whom you also take care of,

word. Finally, he said, "Pat, I will be happy to give Hilda the job. But on one condition. If I like her work, after the strike is over I will keep her. If not, she will come back to manicuring." I extended my hand and we shook on it.

Mr. McLoud knew Hilda's background and hired her as a copywriter in the advertising department, starting her at $60 a week. The strike lasted three months. Afterward, Mr. McLoud came in for his usual daily shave and announced that he was not sending Hilda back to us. He thought she had a good future in advertising. Angelo and I were very happy for Hilda, and so was Hilda!

Within one year, Hilda was making $150 a week, and was offered $300 from Robert Hall Clothes. Under Mr. McLoud's guidance, she took the offer; it would be a few years before she could make as much at Stern's. Everything went well for Hilda. She liked her new job very much. Almost two years later, she received a call from the Marshall Field department store in Chicago, saying that they were interested in her, wanting to speak to her. They offered her $500 a week. Hilda asked our advice. We told her she had to make her own decision. After two weeks of thinking about it, she decided against it, as she would miss the friends she had made in New York City.

After a few years, Hilda was ready for a change. She was making a lot of money, but Robert Hall kept her busy seven days a week. Some nights she even brought work home. She decided to resign and take a part-time job typing, so that she could go back to writing short stories. Her stories were being accepted by *Coronet*. She was fulfilling her ambition.

sent me here. I was going to tell you who I was when you were finished. For recognizing me through the grain of my beard, I will send you two house seats to my show 'Fannie,' with my compliments.''

Suddenly, she discovered that she had cancer. She died of the illness within a year. We heard about Hilda's death from one of our clients who had been recommended to us by Hilda. When he told us, he cried like a baby. Hilda had helped him back from the worst period of his life. She was buried in Middletown, Ohio, leaving everything to her crippled brother.

The barber strike was very rough on Angelo and me. We were working alone and grossing nearly as much as we did with a full crew. Many regular clients wouldn't cross the picket line outside, but new clients came in from other shops. Many of them liked our workmanship and remained clients. Of course, Angelo and I were about forty years old now, and being top-quality barbers didn't do us any harm!

After three months of working very hard, we had had it. We were happy that the strike was over. That is, until our four barbers came in, went to their cabinets, and started packing their tools. We asked them what was going on. Angelo's brother-in-law, Jimmy, and Albert said that they had bought Joe Susca's barbershop across the street, together with another of our

AS FATE WOULD HAVE IT

Henry Morton Robinson was a writer, novelist, and poet. In his book *Water of Life* he referred to moonshine whisky as the water of life. Yet as fate would have it, Henry Morton Robinson died from third-degree burns in his bathtub while drunk in his apartment at the Columbia Club on West Forty-third Street. I lost a good friend, but I also learned a good lesson: Never, never take a bath under the influence of liquor. I still treasure my copy of *Water of Life,* inscribed "To my barber and friend."

barbers, Roger DiSilvestro. They were taking the fourth barber, Pino, with them. When they were all packed, one by one they came to say good-bye. Angelo and I wished them good luck, although I could see the anger in Angelo's eyes because Jimmy had betrayed him. They had taken the telephone numbers of their clients while picketing.

This placed us in a bad situation. Angelo and I discussed whether to call an agency for new barbers or run an ad in a newspaper. Suddenly, George Fedele (the top barber from Joe Susca's shop) came in with his hair disheveled and scratches on his face. He said, "Give me a chair here. I want to work for you two. I will not work for people who have no principles." They insisted that he couldn't leave, holding and pulling him, trying to force him to stay. Imagine our delight—George had almost as large a following as Jimmy, Albert, and Roger put together. (Pino was young and had no following.) George, at thirty-five, was a much more experienced barber than any of them.

After a few days, a barber named Jack Livigni walked in asking for a job. He did not want to go back to a shop where he had worked at Fortieth Street and Madison Avenue. He cited personal reasons. He gave me about one hundred cards of his clients and asked me to call them, as his English was not great. When I called, I found that eight out of ten of them were dead.

He'd had these cards for years! In all, about ten clients came. Jack was an excellent barber, but very slow. We told him not to worry because we had more clients than we could handle. Shortly thereafter, we hired two more barbers through ads in the newspaper. We were now doing more business than we had done before the strike. George often stopped clients from Susca's shop who passed through our lobby. Moreover, a post office adjoined our shop. People were going in and out all day long.

In the meantime, Jimmy, Albert, and Roger had their hands full of problems with the lack of clients at their new shop. A year later, Jimmy and Albert forced Roger to sell his share to them; with three partners, they weren't making enough money. Then they fired Pino for not improving. Pino came to us asking for a job, but we turned him down for being part of the plot to destroy us. We were doing very well. We now had eight barbers and three manicurists. We didn't talk much with Jimmy and Albert, although it was more difficult for Angelo, because Jimmy was his wife's brother.

Tools of the Trade

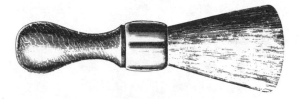

IN the late sixties, innovations began to appear that made honing and stropping razors obsolete. The Schick company came out with the Plus Platinum blade, a disposable razor designed to fit into a regular barber's handle. It was much easier to use and care for than a traditional straight razor, and a professional barber could master it in a comparatively short time. Suddenly, every barber was a good shaver, and every blade was honed to perfection.

Today, most barbers don't even do shaves anymore, and most barbers are called hairstylists anyway. The barbershop—the so-called Man's Kingdom—is gone forever. Here are the cherished tools from that bygone era.

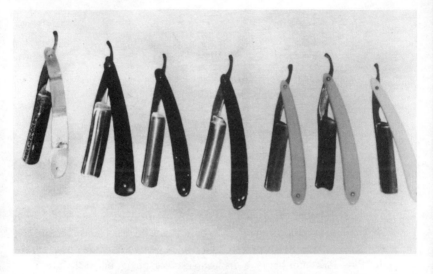

RAZORS

Professional barbers generally preferred razors made in Soliwgen, Germany, although English, French, and Swedish ones were also used. Barbers had a favorite among their razors, choosing the one whose size, shape, and weight best fit their style.

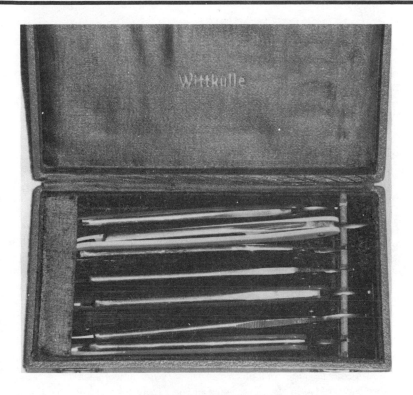

HOME SHAVING BOX

Clients shaving at home usually had a box made to fit seven razors. Each razor was inscribed with one of the days of the week on the handle. Home shavers would bring their set to their barber to hone as needed.

Sharpening Stones

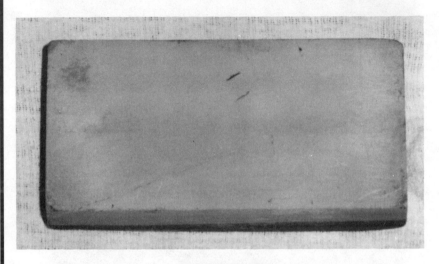

SOAPSTONE

Belgian soapstone has a light cream-colored top and a dark gray bottom. To hone a razor on a soapstone, put shaving lather on the cream-colored side and place the razor, edge side forward, at a slight angle. Glide the blade-edge of the razor along the length of the stone. Turn the blade over and repeat the motion, this time with the edge away from you. Continue for twenty to thirty strokes on each side. To test the edge, run the blade *very lightly* over your thumbnail. When the razor is sharp enough, it will not feel rough as it glides across your nail. A top-notch shaver hones his razors about once a week.

The trick for the barber is to know when a razor is sharp enough to cut the beard and not to feel scratchy or pull. But only 10 percent of professionals ever learn to hone a razor to perfection, as I managed to do. Those barbers who mastered this process were considered the best regardless of their haircutting ability. Clients came in *daily* for shaves and greatly appreciated a barber who didn't cut or hurt them.

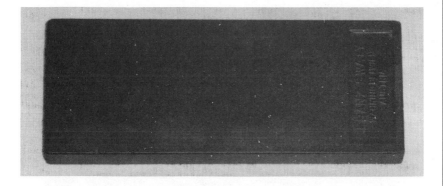

SWATY

Made by Franz Swaty of Beiwien, Austria, this stone is used dry but with the same movement of the razor as on the soapstone. Only three or four strokes are required to put on a good edge, but the blade will only go three shaves between honings. I never mastered the Swaty.

CARBORUNDUM

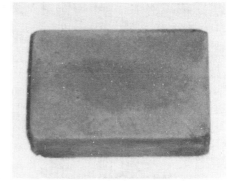

This coarse, domestic stone gives a quick edge to the blade but one that is not quite as sweet on the face. Many barbers compensated for this by processing their Carborundum stones to make them smoother and sweeter. The barber covers the stone with Vaseline, wraps it in a towel, and places it in a steam sterilizer for a couple of hours. Once processed, the stone lasts for years. My stone was first processed in 1929 by a barber I worked with, and I used it until my retirement in 1982. I could get twelve shaves out of one honing (four strokes per side) and get as sweet an edge as from the soapstone.

THE RAZOR STROP

After honing, a razor must be stropped to give the ultimate smoothness to the edge. A strop has a smooth-finished leather strip on one side and a heavy piece of linen on the other. Usually about 18 inches long by 3 inches wide, the strop is attached by a hook under the right armrest of the barber's chair. Begin with the linen side and finish with the leather to impart the sweetest edge. To use, drag the razor from the hook to the handle with the edge away from you. Flip the razor over and go back up. But if the razor isn't honed properly first, the stropping won't do any good!

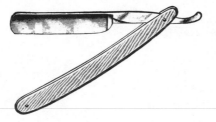

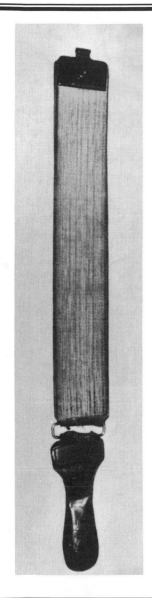

The Razor Strop
(linen side)

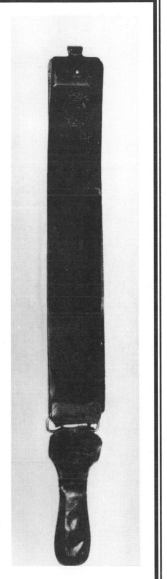

The Razor Strop
(leather side)

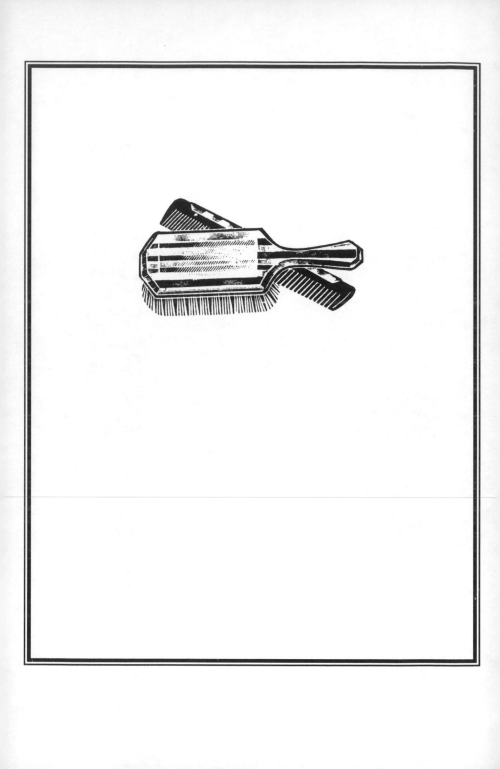

7

FROM 1941 to 1945, because of the war, we had not had any mail from Sicily. Although my parents trusted my Uncle Francesco with the properties he was looking after, they decided to take a trip to Licodia Eubea to analyze the situation. The family still thought of moving back to Sicily, always thinking of the good life they could have there.

On their arrival, Uncle Francesco was very attentive to them. One day, Uncle Nunzio, my mother's other brother, who had been jealous of the power we had given Francesco, whispered into my father's ear, "Come to my house tomorrow at ten. I want to talk to you alone." My father nodded. Next morning, my father told my mother and Uncle Francesco that he was going to the bank on some private business and would return in an hour.

Uncle Nunzio told my father about Uncle Francesco's behavior during our absence. Our house had been lent to the man in charge of buying all produce and grain for the Fascist government—for no rent! He

ART LOGEN, MEN'S MODEL

Art Logen was sent to me by a model agency that sent me all its models for haircuts before photography sessions. They gave me written specifications on the style of haircut, but they left the particulars to my discretion.

During the fall of 1963, Art and I began to talk about the stock market. It was a favorite topic in the barbershop. I had officers of many large companies as clients, and occasionally they gave me stock tips that I passed along to other clients, who reciprocated by giving me tips on their companies. During this period, I couldn't take advantage of my information. I had married off two of my three daughters, but had one more to go.

By the end of 1963, Art, taking advantage of my tips, had done very well. They were all winners. In early 1964, we decided to keep track of his investments based on my tips. At the end of the year, he had made a profit of more than $100,000 on my

allowed Uncle Francesco to sell 10 percent of the produce and grain to the government and the remaining 90 percent at black market prices, five times higher than government-controlled prices. The money Uncle Francesco made from this was never deposited in the bank; he hid the money in the house. Furthermore uncle Francesco made private loans to people with this money at 20 percent interest. He was ruthless in his business dealings and was hated by everyone in the town. People avoided him. He had lost all his friends, and the family had nothing to do with him.

My father wanted to take Uncle Francesco to court for misrepresentation and maladministration. The family, as much as they were against him, realized he would be fined and receive a heavy jail sentence. They talked my father out of it. Instead uncle Francesco had to pay $5,000 for maladministration of our property and was stripped of all our properties. It didn't make any difference to him, as he had become very wealthy. When he died, we heard that no one offered to carry his casket, which is customary of friends and relatives, everyone following the funeral procession to the cemetery at the edge of town.

Men had to be hired to carry the casket.

My parents were outraged, and also disappointed. They had been taken in by a man whom we trusted implicity. Worse, he was family, a man I had looked up to as a father since childhood and who loved me as a son. I suppose greed can push someone to do the unthinkable. My parents now abandoned the idea of moving back to Licodia Eubea. Land there was now worth less than we had paid for it, because no one was farming. Most young men had emigrated to West Germany, Northern Italy, Australia, and the United States. They rented our lands for what they could get and waited for a seller's market.

We were in America to stay, having cut our roots to the old country. I'll always miss the beautiful lands of Sicily, but at least I've always had the good fortune to enjoy my favorite Italian pastime in this country—small-game hunting! Through the generosity of my clients and friends, some of the beautiful lands around New York City have been open for me to hunt game on. Many of my best memories come from days hunting on these lands, and I'll always remember with fondness the wonderful days I spent with the best dogs a person

information. One day in 1965, he came in and beckoned me to follow him to the back of the shop. Excusing myself to my client, I followed him to see what he had in mind. Pulling out a check from his shirt pocket, he said, "I know you have no money to invest. Here is $10,000. I want you to buy whatever stock you want with the verbal understanding that if you make money, you keep the profit and give me back the $10,000. If you lose, I will absorb the loss. Also I want to know what stock you buy so I can buy some myself." I was flabbergasted. I thanked him profusely and immediately told him that I was going to buy Maxon Electronics at $10 per share.

During the first week, Maxon went up to $11.50. Art called me twice from his new home in Spring Lake, New Jersey, offering me more money. I said, "No, you have done enough." At the end of three months, I sold the stock, making a $4,000 profit. I bought a new car and sent Art $10,000, thanking him very much. Art kept his stock for six months for a long-term profit, making $25,000 for himself.

WARD MELVILLE

Ward Melville was chairman of the board of the Melville Shoe Corporation and benefactor of the town of Stony Brook, Long Island. Angelo and I met Mr. Melville when we bought the Arcade Barber Shop. He was an unusually fine gentleman, soft-spoken, humane, humble, and a great philanthropist. He was responsible for the success of Thom McAn Shoes, which eventually grew into a conglomerate, the Melville Shoe Corporation.

Mr. Melville had a beautiful estate at Old Field Point, near Stony Brook. He knew my love of small-game hunting with beagles, so he gave me permission to hunt on all lands owned by him and the Suffolk Improvement Company of Stony Brook and Old Field. I had the best hunting of my life there with my dad and friends of mine, until he donated the

could dream of. This is a story about one of them: Buddy.

In 1960, my beagle hound, McKenzie's Duke, was ten years old (the life expectancy of a hunting dog is about twelve years). I decided to mate him, hoping to get a son to replace him when his time came. If I was lucky, his son would have the opportunity to hunt with him for a couple of years and learn the tricks of the rabbit to elude the dog. Duke knew them all. He was mated to Bronx Beauty. After sixty-three days, they were the proud parents of a litter of seven, four males and three females. I chose a male who was the image of his father both in color and build. I named him "Pat's Buddy."

He was both intelligent and good-natured. By three months, he learned to retrieve to perfection, bringing the canvas training dummy gently, so as not to damage the game. Soon he was hunting alongside his father and learning very fast. He loved to hunt. By the age of one, I had taught him to stop with one blast of my whistle. He would look up at me and obey my hand signal without my saying a word.

One Saturday morning I took him to train at Howard Beach. There was much open land there, alive with rabbits and pheasants. While chasing a rabbit, and barking continuously (as dogs do when they are on the scent of game), he gave an agonized yelp. I ran to him and found that he had cut his leg on a broken milk bottle. After I tied his leg with my handkerchief to stop the bleeding, I carried him to my car and drove him to Dr. Campagnine, a vet on Flatbush Avenue. It took fifteen stitches to close the wound, and two of Buddy's nerves had been cut by the glass. He took a month to heal. Because of the cut nerves, his foot remained flat instead of erect when standing, but it bothered him only on a hard day's hunt.

During a hunt, we usually had two, three, or four dogs, but Buddy was the one we depended on most. He was always the leader. If one of the hunters had a rabbit jump in front of him and couldn't get a shot at it because of heavy underbrush, he would yell "Coniglio" (meaning rabbit in Italian) to let the other hunters know that a rabbit was on the run. They would stop and keep still so that if the rabbit went in their direction, they wouldn't be seen. Hopefully, the hunter would see the rabbit as it ran and have the opportunity to shoot. After hearing the yell "Coniglio" on about a dozen hunting trips, Buddy came to under-

land to the state for a university. It was excellent for grouse, pheasant, quail, and rabbits.

One story stands out in my mind about Mr. Melville. One day, he came in without an appointment for a fast shave. I was busy, so he sat in one of the other barbers' chairs. No one had ever shaved him in our shop except my partner Angelo and me. His beard would lie down as it came out of the skin, and unless the skin was stretched, the razor would glide over his beard with only soap coming off. I warned the barber. He put the lather on the beard, and while rubbing (he rubbed more than usual, hoping to soften the beard more), Mr. Melville said, "It's not going to come off by rubbing it." The barber proceeded to shave him, but he had not stretched the skin enough, so the blade picked up only the lather and not the beard. He changed direction with the razor, making it painful and making the skin bleed, changing razors as he went but with the same results. The barber was both embarrassed and perspiring. Tears were coming out of Mr. Melville's eyes. Finally, the barber finished the ordeal. He was humiliated. Mr. Melville gave him double the usual tip and told him, "It was a fine shave." He knew the barber had tried his best with his problem beard. Mr. Melville never spoke about this incident to me. It was typical of him.

Every June, the Melvilles went to their beautiful estate, Wide Water, in Old Field Point. Mr. Melville was meticulous about his hair and didn't like the haircuts given to him by Stony Brook barbers.

One summer day I went to visit one of my daughters who was now married and living in Selden, Long Island. I brought my barber tools to cut my son-in-law's hair. While there, I remembered that Mr. Melville had not shown up at the shop for two weeks, so I called him, telling him that I was nearby and would be glad to go to Wide Water to give him a trim. He was very grateful. When I arrived, the maid

stand its meaning. He would run to the hunter that yelled and practically ask the hunter, "Which way did it go?" The hunter would put his hand to the ground and drag it in the direction the rabbit had fled. Buddy would follow with his nose to the ground and within seconds would be on the scent, barking after the rabbit. The other dogs, upon hearing Buddy, would join in the chase, all barking together, making music for the hunters. The rabbit would run from three hundred to one thousand feet, depending on the speed of the dogs following the scent, unless he dove into his hole. Eventually, the rabbit would turn back to his starting point. The hunters, knowing this, would be waiting about fifty feet apart for the kill. They would wait for the dogs to see the dead rabbit and then start searching for the next one. Buddy, one of the few beagles to learn to retrieve, would pick up the rabbit and bring it happily to the nearest hunter who called him by name.

Buddy continued to improve. Some years earlier, Ward Melville had given me permission to hunt on all the lands owned by him and the Suffolk Improvement Company in and around Stony Brook. Of all these lands, the best hunting was on the grounds on which the State University of New York at Stony Brook now stands. It was excellent for pheasant, quail, partridge, and rabbits.

Many times while hunting there, we would also watch a foxhunt going on simultaneously. The foxhounds would follow a scent made with a piece of canvas saturated with fox scent and dragged on paths through the woods. The path would end on a road where cars would be waiting for the hunters, all dressed in red jackets for the hunt. There was also a van for the foxhounds to bring them back to their kennels for feeding at Mrs. Melville's estate, Wide Water, at Old Field Point.

One Sunday, my friends Phil Guglielmino, Vincent Modica, and I went for a day's hunt with Buddy and Vincent's fine dog, Duke. (He was a brother of Buddy and named after his father.) We heard the horn of the hunt master starting the foxhunt and putting the dogs on the scent. Within seconds, the twenty or so foxhounds were barking after the scent as the hunters on horseback followed them. We always stopped hunting until they passed. But this time, their lead dog went off the trail to follow the scent of

led me to the terrace, where I cut Mr. Melville's hair. The terrace was large, with a beautiful view of Long Island Sound and the Connecticut coastline.

When I was about to leave, Mr. Melville handed me $20 and thanked me. I said, "Mr. Melville, since 1947, thanks to you, I've had the best hunting of my life here. Many times I wanted to do something for you but could never think how. Coming here today to cut your hair has solved my problem. I would gladly come during the summer when you can't come to the shop. But if you insist on paying me, I will never come here again to cut your hair." Mr. Melville said, "If you feel that way, I would appreciate your calling me when I delay. Thank you very much."

In the fall of 1971, Mr. Melville had a stroke that left him in a wheelchair and almost blind. He was able to see only shadows. He was brought to the shop a few times by his nurse. I made a tape with my mandolin, announcing each song, and sent it to him.

In June, they went, as usual, to Wide Water for the summer. On my first visit to give him a haircut, Mrs. Melville said, "Now that we know that you play the mandolin, how about giving us a private concert?" I said I would be delighted. So, through that summer, every two weeks, after cutting Mr. Melville's hair, we sat on the terrace and I played for an hour with Mrs. Melville singing along with me. During the concerts, one of their maids served homemade goodies and drinks.

At the end of the summer, after the usual mandolin concert, while we enjoyed a drink together, Mr. Melville asked if I had thought of where I wanted to retire when my working days were over. I had never given it a thought, but I said that it would be in this area, because my three daughters had bought homes near here. Then he said, "I would like to help you buy a retirement home."

The following Saturday morning, I received a call from a man telling me that he

a real fox. He ran straight toward us. Buddy and Duke, seeing the foxhounds, ran away. Buddy and Duke split. So did the hounds. Duke sped by me, and I ran in front of the foxhounds waving my arms and yelling, trying to scare them off. They turned to join the others who were pursuing Buddy. After a few frantic minutes, we saw Buddy limping back with difficulty. We ran to him and saw that they had ripped his stomach and his behind.

Suddenly, we heard the hounds coming to finish him off. Picking up Buddy with my left hand, I told Jimmy and Vincent to shoot in the air when I gave the word. As they came within one hundred feet of us, my hunting partners started shooting their shotguns. The hounds, not used to shotgun blasts, turned and ran. I carried Buddy to the car and circled the road until we found where the foxhunt was supposed to end. We were told that the hunt would soon be over and that a veterinarian was among the hunters. I soon met Dr. Fredricks, who, upon seeing Buddy's condition, told me to bring him immediately to his hospital in Huntington. Once there, he suggested that we leave Buddy in his care. In sixty days the wound healed completely, and

Buddy continued to hunt for years afterward.

One weekend, my friend Flavio Mascera and I decided to hunt the property of a friend of mine in Surprise, New York. The owner of the property was Vincent Gramm, a professor of languages in Albany. Flavio had his dog Junie and I had Buddy, who was now twelve and one-half years old. He looked and hunted like a five-year old. We hunted Saturday, bagging ten rabbits and four partridges. On Sunday morning, after two hours of hunting, we shot three rabbits and one partridge. Buddy was chasing a rabbit toward me when suddenly I heard him give an agonized yelp. I ran over and found him dead. He had a heart attack. It was a black day for me and my friend, Flavio. I went to the house to get a shovel. Mrs. Gramm came back with me. She dug the grave for Buddy as Flavio and I were too stunned to dig. I hunted there until 1982 and always visited Buddy's grave.

was a retired lawyer, a friend of Mr. Melville, and Mr. Melville had assigned him to help me find a home for my retirement. He asked if I could come out that day; he had something to show me. Connie and I made an appointment to meet him at the Stony Brook railroad station at noon. On our arrival, after introducing ourselves, we got in his car. He said, "Let me tell you what Mr. Melville has in mind for you. He will give you $20,000 to put toward the purchase of a house." He added, "If I were you, I wouldn't waste too much time on this. If anything happens to Mr. Melville, you will lose everything." We thanked him very much for his trouble and his advice. Four days later, he called my daughter Katherine, to show her a house on Terryville Road. We liked the house and bought it, paying the difference above $20,000.

8

ON September 9, 1967, *The New Yorker* came out with another story about our shop.

TIES

Charity is said to begin at home, and so, on occasion, does journalism. We have a story to tell you about the Arcade Barber Shop, here in the lobby of our building. The shop is a pleasant, convivial spot, with a clientele more varied and distinguished than its modest setting would suggest (among the regular patrons are Alec Waugh, Vincent Sardi, Jr., State Senator Jack E. Bronston, and Johnny Carson), but what chiefly interests us about it is the fact that of its seven barbers no fewer than four came from the same small town in Sicily. The majority of the barbers in the city are Italians, and of this majority a large fraction are Sicilians, who have been famous over the centuries for the close ties to family and place of origin that they are able to maintain, however formidable the barriers of time and distance, and thus it happens—no doubt to the bewilderment of a new customer—that the ordinary round of events in a remote and impoverished little town in the mountains of Sicily daily becomes the subject of animated discussion from chair to chair in this barber shop in midtown Manhattan.

The name of the town is Licodia Eubea, and it stands on an elevation of some two thousand feet thirty-five miles inland from the port city of Catania. It is a pretty town, the barbers say, with narrow, winding streets, stone houses roofed with red tiles, and, at its highest point, the ruins of an ancient fortified castle tumbled long ago by an earthquake; from time to time, diggers into the ruins have exposed whole rooms of the castle, still furnished as they were when the earthquake struck. The main products of the countryside around Licodia Eubea are wheat, oranges, lemons, grapes, and olives; in the old feudal fashion, the farmers live in the town and have to spend a considerable part of every day getting to and from their fields and orchards. The town used to be prosperous, but the farms are no longer profitable, and for decades the young people have been moving away, not only to the United States but also to northern Italy, and to Switzerland, Germany, and Australia.

The first of the barbers to leave Licodia Eubea was one of its two owners, Pat—short for Pasquale—Spagnuolo. (The other owner, Angelo Copertino, comes from Bari, on the Adriatic, but he says that in the twenty-two years he and Pat have owned the Arcade he has come to feel like a native of Licodia and sometimes hears himself using words of Licodian dialect.) Pat, who was born in Licodia in 1911, came to this country with his parents in 1920; having married the daughter of a Licodian, he returned to Licodia with her, and with his parents, in 1933, expecting to run the family farm there. Mussolini's sword-rattling caused the Spagnuolos to fear that war was imminent, however, so after only a year they came back to New York. Pat held on to the farm until last year, and then sold it only because he had come to realize that the longer he owned it the less it would be worth. Felice Guglielmino, known in the shop as Phil, was born in Licodia in 1929 and left in 1948. When, at the outbreak of the Second World War, the Licodia barbers were drafted, little Felice boldly took up barbering, learning the trade from an uncle and practicing with the help of a large wooden box to stand on. Having left Licodia, Phil nevertheless took care to marry a Licodian girl; so did Rosario—nicknamed Sal—Aliotta, who was born in Licodia in 1931, came here in 1955, and in 1959, made a trip to Licodia expressly to acquire a bride. The fourth Arcade barber from Licodia is Vito Nobile, who was born in 1946, moved to this country with his parents in 1959, and married a Licodian girl back in Licodia in 1965.

Pat, Phil, Sal, and Vito keep in close touch with Licodia and, like all Licodians, sometimes speculate about going back there to live when they are old. "I think maybe I would have been as happy there as here," Pat says. "It is hard to believe how different the life there is."

During all my years of barbering, I made sure to keep up with my musical interests. After returning from Sicily for the last time, I didn't have many opportunities to serenade beautiful young women for their amorous suitors, but I managed to keep in practice. Occasionally, if I didn't have a client waiting, I would pick up my mandolin or violin and play for whoever was in the shop. It was an extra part of the Arcade Barber Shop's expert service!

One day in 1968, my wife's brother, Dr. Thomas DiMartino, brought his wife and six children to meet their family in New York City. Connie and I invited them over for dinner, and during the meal my brother-in-law told me that his son John wanted to take up the violin. He wondered where he could buy a violin that wouldn't be too expensive.

After dinner, thinking about things, I realized that I had not played my violin in quite a while. My wife had become manic-depressive since the accidental death of our granddaughter years ago. During Connie's illness, I lost the will to play, and my violin had sat unused in the basement for two years. I couldn't let that go on.

Later on, I struck up a conversation with my young nephew John and asked him about his ambition to play the violin. He was very enthusiastic. He told me that since his mother played piano and his father sang, he wanted to be a part of it all. Delighted, I took him to the basement and showed him my violin, the one I had played since I was eleven years old. "I'm giving you my violin," I said. "Take care of it, and learn to play well."

In 1971, after seven years of suffering, my wife and I heard about Dr. Seymour Rosenblatt. On her first visit to him, Dr. Rosenblatt placed Connie on Lithium (then a relatively new medication). In three days, she was so much improved I thought it was a miracle. She got better and better with each passing day.

About six months later, a much-recovered Connie asked me why I didn't play the violin any longer and only played the mandolin. I told her about giving the violin to John, and, much to my surprise, she became angry. She wanted me to call her brother and have him return the violin. Since I felt I couldn't do that, I promised to get a new instrument.

Later that week, Martin Mayer (a client for twenty

years) came to me for his usual biweekly haircut. As he was a noted music critic and writer and knew many people in the music industry, I explained my awful situation to him and asked him if he could help me find a new violin. He said, "It's funny that you should ask me. A few years ago, a violin teacher convinced me that he could teach me to play in six months or less. So, I bought a violin for about $500 and started taking lessons. After taking lessons for over six months, I came to the conclusion that I could never learn to play the violin well. I stopped taking lessons and put the violin in a closet where it has sat ever since. If you want me to bring it in for you to try it tomorrow, I will."

I told him I would love to try it, and the next day he brought it to me. He said that when he returned from an upcoming ten-day lecture tour, he would see me again.

I liked his violin very much. It was a little larger than mine, but it had a beautiful tone. When Mr. Mayer came back for his next haircut, I asked for the price, unless of course he would care to give it to me. He laughed, but on his next visit he offered the violin to me as a gift. My wife was thrilled to hear me playing and practicing daily.

About a year later, Roger DiMartino, another brother-in-law, went to visit Thomas and his family. During the visit, he saw a violin that no one seemed to play. Asking his brother about it, Roger found out that it belonged to John, who had given it up after two years of lessons. No one played it now.

Roger, who played many instruments but none of them well, asked if he could take it. On our next visit to Roger's house, he told Connie and me about his new violin. I naturally suspected it to be mine. Upon seeing it, I recognized it as the one I had played since I was a child. I told Roger the whole story, and he was more than happy to return it to me. But now I had two violins.

On the day of his next visit to my shop, I brought Martin Mayer's violin in. As he sat in the barber's chair for his haircut, I told him, "Martin, my violin came back home, and I'm returning yours with thanks and gratitude."

He was very surprised and said "Now it goes back in the closet. Who knows? Maybe someday I'll take it up again."

The Arcade Barber Shop had smooth sailing until 1970, when Angelo, my partner of twenty-six years, decided to sell his share in the business and retire to Boynton Beach, Florida. His wife needed a warmer climate.

He recommended his clients to the other six barbers in the shop, as I was very busy with the clientele I had built up ever since 1935, but a few insisted on my taking care of them. One of these was Joseph Wolf, who had been a faithful client of Angelo's since 1929. He was a C.P.A. and came to Manhattan twice a week from Brooklyn to see his clients. He always called Angelo for an appointment a day or two before his usual haircut, shave, and massage. He was always a half hour early for his appointment. He would put his briefcase on the hat rack and say, "I'm going to Schrafft's for an ice-cream soda. I'll be back in half an hour."

The second time I took care of him, he said apologetically, "Pat, why is it that Angelo gave me an hour of his time, and you give me only forty-five minutes?" What he didn't know was that during the massage, when Angelo had three Turkish towels over his face with only his nose showing during the witch hazel steam, and Mr. Wolf was snoring, Angelo would go to the luncheonette next door, have coffee and cake, and come back in fifteen minutes. Mr. Wolf never missed him. Of course, I couldn't tell him that, so I just said that I worked faster than Angelo. If he wanted a slower barber, I suggested Jack Livigni. Jack would take an hour and twenty-five minutes. Mr. Wolf said, "No, I like the way you work." He never mentioned the subject again, and I never revealed Angelo's secret.

Benny Monticciolo, one of our barbers for about ten years, begged me to let him buy Angelo's share. I gave his proposal much thought. Since I was nearing sixty-five and didn't want added responsibility, I agreed. Benny asked me to run the shop, since he had no managerial experience. He would work on the chair. All went well for two and a half years, until Benny, wanting to change the fixtures, also wanted to add women barbers, thus creating a unisex barbershop. I was against it. A unisex shop would drive away our old clientele, who were accustomed to a men's barbershop. If the shop hadn't been doing well, I would have gone along with Benny, but the shop was doing very well.

Benny and I continued together for another year, but we were not happy with each other. Moreover, my mother was ill with cancer, and my wife Connie had also been ill since 1964. The problems with Benny became intolerable. After a year of these bad feelings, I decided to sell him the shop, as I was nearing sixty-five years old. I valued the shop at $30,000, but he told me that according to friends, half a share was worth no more than $10,000. Analyzing the situation, I felt that the only advantage he had on me was his age, and I decided to offer him the shop for $15,000. He refused, and

I immediately said that I'd buy it from him for $15,000. He said okay. When I started to call my lawyer to draw up the papers, Benny said that he wanted until the next morning to think it over.

The next morning, Benny said, "Why can't we stay as we are?" I said, "Nothing doing. Either you buy it or I will," forcing him to make the decision to buy. Immediately I made him come with me to our lawyer to draw up the contract. This was in July 1975, and the terms of the contract would not become final until December 31, 1976.

As 1976 progressed, Benny and I became more unhappy with each other. Benny found it agonizing to wait to make the changes in the shop that he had planned. In the meantime, I had to decide what I would do after selling Benny the shop. Around June, I decided to rent a chair in the Graybar Building barbershop at 420 Lexington Avenue, working Tuesday, Wednesday, and Thursday, from nine to four. According to our contract, Benny and I must be separated by five blocks north or south and three avenues east or west of the Arcade Barber Shop.

I decided to offer the shop to Benny on October 1, 1976, instead of the end of the year, provided that he allowed me to tell only my clients where I was going. He immediately agreed.

Other barbers in the shop told me that Benny didn't think many clients would follow me, especially with my working only Tuesday, Wednesday, and Thursday and being three avenues away.

I had to work out an alternative. As eventually, on retirement, I would move to Long Island to be near my three daughters, I told all my clients who lived on

Long Island and played golf that I was interested in getting a concession in a golf club to work Wednesday, Saturday, and Sunday, the busiest days at any golf club. Among the clients who took it upon themselves to get me some information was Professor Julius C. Edelstein, the Dean at City College, across the street from the shop. Although he didn't play golf, his close and good friend ex-Mayor Robert Wagner did, and he was influential at the Sands Point Golf Club. The Dean promised to speak to him about me. A short time after that, as I was crossing Forty-third Street on my way home, I spotted ex-Mayor Wagner. I approached him and introduced myself as Professor Edelstein's barber. He immediately said, "Yes, Professor Edelstein spoke to me about you." He mentioned that any barber having a concession in a good golf club would rarely give it up, but he said he would look into it. He asked for my telephone number at home and said that if anything came up on the matter, he would call me.

On October 1, I moved to my new location. To my amazement, all my clientele followed me. Three months later Wagner called me at home to tell me that the opportunity at the golf club had arrived. I thanked him very much, telling him that since all my clients had followed me, I had decided to stay with them. He said, "You're doing the right thing."

I did very well for two years. Then the stipulation that I work five blocks from the Arcade was now over, and I began looking around for a location near the old shop to make it easier for my clients. When Benny heard about this, he called me, saying that he wanted to meet me that evening at home. (We lived only three doors from each other.) He offered me a bigger percentage than what I was getting, saying that after working thirty-one years at the Arcade, I belonged there. I told him I would let him know my decision the next day.

In the morning, I came to the conclusion that it was easier to bring my clients to the Arcade than to a new shop. I spoke with Benny again that evening, making him promise that he was on the up-and-up and that there were no schemes. He swore that I would be my own boss and whatever help I could give, he'd appreciate. On returning to the Arcade, my clients were delighted, particularly because it was much closer to their offices. But it was not the same shop. It was noisy and disorderly. I noticed that the clientele was different. It didn't bother me since I worked exclusively on my own clients. I worked three days a week at a barber chair in the rear of the shop. As time went on, the shop began to get worse.

After two years, he sold the shop to someone named Frank, who also owned a shop across the street on Forty-third Street. Not knowing his ability to run the shop, I decided to leave. I spoke to Louis, the owner of the Leftcourt Barber Shop at 521 Fifth Avenue, on the corner of Forty-third Street (this was the shop that Barney Penn had offered to let me manage in 1941). He offered me a chair in a booth, with equal conditions. I accepted his offer, and waited until Benny contracted for the sale of the shop before I told him. The new owner rebelled, begging me to remain and offering me any chair and better conditions. I felt sorry for him. He had bought the shop including my business. Benny tried hard to convince me to stay, particularly because things looked bad for him. But my mind was made up, and I moved to the booth at 521 Fifth Avenue.

I was treated very well there by Louis, whom I had known for almost fifteen years. And, as usual, my clients followed me. They liked the privacy of the booth. It seemed like my own little shop.

After two years, it became obvious that I had to retire, because of Connie's health. So, on August 1, 1982, I ended a barbering career of fifty-five years. Most of my clients had been with me from twenty to forty-eight years, following me from shop to shop, and I felt obligated to place each one with a barber who would give him quality workmanship. I also wanted to give each one a barber near his office.

I had approximately one hundred clients. I picked three barbers from different locations: Joseph Nicotra at Forty-ninth Street and Fifth Avenue; Enzo Curti at the Arcade Barber Shop; and Jimmy Liali at the Graybar Barber Shop. Then I prepared three little telephone books, giving each barber a book with the names of the clients I was recommending to him, and after each name, what the client usually wanted plus any peculiarities that he had. I wanted each client to feel at ease with his new barber. I met with the three one evening each and we went over the lists. I told all of them that I was recommending these clients to them because I felt they possessed the qualities to please them. This was the very least I could do. They were more than clients, they were my friends. I wanted nothing else than to have pleased the client to make my fifty-five-year barbering career complete.

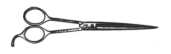

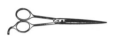 ## MY GOLDEN RULES OF
SERVING THE PUBLIC

1. Smile at the person you are to attend and mean it. Look him straight in the eye and give the impression that you are happy to be of service.
2. Always be neat looking. At no time neglect how you look. You will be respected accordingly.
3. Never use only your first name. If you do, you degrade yourself. Use your last name, as it lends you more respect.
4. Never call a client by his first name unless he asks you to.
5. Never speak to someone at a short distance. Be aware of the possibility of bad breath, and in addition to bathing regularly, use deodorant.
6. Always be punctual for appointments.
7. Always memorize people's preferences. Don't make them tell you what they want over and over. If necessary, put facts about clients next to their names in your telephone book.
8. Never speak another language while you are working on a client, even if you ask permission.

9. Always be fair with your co-workers, otherwise they will gang up to make you miserable.
10. If you are not as fast as your co-workers, don't work faster to keep up with them, because your work will suffer. Instead, do your very best at your natural speed. The employer who hired you doesn't expect you to rush through your work. He's obviously happy with the way you are, or you wouldn't be employed there.
11. Never ask clients personal questions. If they want to, they will tell you about themselves, particularly when you have gained their confidence.
12. If a regular client talks about his family, remember it. Always ask him about his family.
13. If a client keeps his sideburns straight, always has a close shave, or keeps his mustache trimmed, compliment him, telling him that very few clients do that. Everyone likes to be praised. If he needs your suggestions, offer them. You will find that the client will have more confidence in you if you make suggestions for other services you believe would be beneficial to him.
14. As an employer, if you want an employee to respect the morning starting time, you must also respect his quitting time in the evening.
15. An employer must always be an example to his employees of the dos and don'ts in the shop. He must practice his good habits and tactfully overcome the bad habits of his employees.
16. Never play favorites. If you do, keep it to yourself (just as a father keeps secret his favorites among his children).